Twenty Years of Health System Reform in Brazil

DIRECTIONS IN DEVELOPMENT
Human Development

Twenty Years of Health System Reform in Brazil

An Assessment of the Sistema Único de Saúde

Michele Gragnolati, Magnus Lindelow, and Bernard Couttolenc

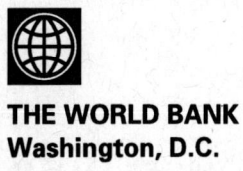

THE WORLD BANK
Washington, D.C.

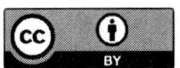

Contents

Boxes

Figures

Tables

About the Authors

Michele Gragnolati is the Human Development Sector Leader for Argentina, Paraguay, and Uruguay at the World Bank, based in Buenos Aires. Previously, he served as Human Development Sector Leader for Brazil, based in Brasilia; human development country sector coordinator for the Western Balkans, based in Sarajevo; and human development economist, based in Washington, DC. He holds a bachelor's degree in economics from Bocconi University in Milan, a master of science degree in demography from the London School of Economics, and a doctorate in statistical demography from Princeton University.

Magnus Lindelow is the Human Development Sector Leader (Health, Education, and Social Protection) at the World Bank in Brazil. He holds a doctorate in economics from Oxford University. At the World Bank, he has worked on health system reform, service delivery, public expenditure management, and poverty and social protection issues. Over the last few years, he has been involved in projects and research in Cambodia, China, the Lao People's Democratic Republic, Malaysia, Mongolia, the Republic of the Union of Myanmar, Thailand, Timor-Leste, and, most recently, Brazil. He has published books and research articles on impact evaluation of health sector programs, distributional issues in the health sector, public finance, service delivery, poverty, and other topics. Prior to joining the World Bank, he worked as an economist in the Ministry of Planning and Finance in Mozambique and later as a consultant on public finance and health sector issues.

Bernard Couttolenc is Chief Executive Officer of the Performa Institute, a new policy research center in São Paulo, Brazil. He has a master's degree in business management and a doctorate in health economics from Johns Hopkins University. He has worked for many years in executive positions in public and private hospitals in Brazil as well as in planning and financing of the public health system. He has nearly 20 years of experience consulting with international organizations such as the Asian Development Bank, Inter-American Development Bank, World Bank, and World Health Organization, among others. He has participated in projects in 15 developing countries in Africa, Asia, and Latin America on health sector reform; health financing and payment mechanisms; hospital management, efficiency and reform; health care financing; health systems planning and evaluation; and public-private partnerships. For more than 10 years, he held a teaching position at the University of São Paulo, where he conducted research in health economics, financing, and economic evaluation.

Abbreviations

AIH	*autorização de internação hospitalar,* the inpatient care information and billing system of the SUS
AMS	Assistência Médico-Sanitária, a survey by the IBGE
ANS	Agência Nacional de Saúde Suplementar, National Regulatory Agency for Private Health Insurance and Plans
BRICS	five upper-middle-income emerging countries: Brazil, Russia, India, China, and (recently) South Africa
CNI	Confederação Nacional da Indústria, National Confederation of Industry
CONASS	Conselho Nacional de Secretários de Saúde, National Council of State Secretaries of Health
CPMF	Contribuição Provisória sobre Movimentações Financeiras, a contribution of financial transactions passed to finance the public health system
CT	computerized tomography
DATASUS	data-processing arm of the Ministry of Health
ESF	Family Health Strategy
GAPA	Grupo de Apoio à Prevenção à AIDS
GDP	gross domestic product
HIV/AIDS	human immunodeficiency virus/acquired immunodeficiency syndrome
IBGE	Instituto Brasileiro de Geografia e Estatística, Brazilian Institute of Geography and Statistics
IDSUS	Índice de Desempenho do SUS, SUS Performance Indicator
INAMPS	Instituto Nacional de Assistência Médica da Previdência Social, National Institute for Social Medical Assistance, in charge of curative care under the Social Security system that preceded SUS
IPEA	Instituto de Pesquisa Econômica Aplicada, Institute of Applied Economic Research
MAC	*média e alta complexidade,* a grouping of medium- and high-complexity services in SUS classification of health care levels

	and a block grant covering most inpatient care and specialized care
MRI	magnetic resonance imaging
OECD	Organisation for Economic Co-operation and Development
PACS	Programa de Agentes Comunitários de Saúde, Community Health Agents Program that preceded the ESF
PMAQ	Programa Nacional de Melhoria do Acesso e da Qualidade da Atenção Básica, National Program for Improvement of Access and Quality in Primary Care
PNAD	Pesquisa Nacional por Amostra de Domicílios, IBGE's yearly household survey
POF	Pesquisa dos Orçamentos Familiares, a household survey
PROCON	Bureau of Consumer Protection
SAMU	Sistema de Assistência Médica de Urgência, Mobile Emergency Service
SIOPS	Sistema de Informação sobre Orçamentos Públicos em Saúde, Public Health Budget Information System of the Ministry of Health, which records and monitors budgetary expenditures on health from all levels of government
SUDS	Unified and Decentralized Health System
SUS	Sistema Único de Saúde, Unified Health System
TCU	Tribunal de Contas da União
WHO	World Health Organization

Overview

It has been more than 20 years since the 1988 Constitution formally established the Brazilian Unified Health System (Sistema Único de Saúde, SUS). The impetus for the SUS came in part from rising costs and a crisis in the Social Security system that preceded the reforms, but also from a broad-based political movement calling for democratization and improved social rights. Building on reforms that started in the 1980s, the SUS was based on three overarching principles: (a) universal access to health services, with health defined as a citizen's right and an obligation of the state; (b) equality of access to health care; and (c) integrality (comprehensiveness) and continuity of care. Other guiding ideas included decentralization, increased participation, and evidence-based prioritization (Couttolenc 2011a).

The SUS reforms established health as a fundamental right and duty of the state and started a process of fundamentally transforming Brazil's health system to achieve this goal. This report focuses on two questions: What has been achieved since the SUS was established? And what challenges remain in achieving the goals that were established in 1988? The report assesses whether the SUS reforms have transformed the health system as envisaged more than 20 years ago and whether the reforms have led to improved outcomes with regard to access to services, financial protection, and health status.

Any effort to assess performance confronts a host of challenges concerning the definition of boundaries of the "health system," the outcomes that the assessment should focus on, the sources and quality of data, and the role of policies and reforms in explaining how the performance of the health system has changed over time. Building on an extensive literature on health system assessment, this report is based on a simple framework that specifies a set of "building blocks" that affect intermediate outcomes such as access, quality, and efficiency, which, in turn, contribute to final outcomes, including health status, financial protection, and satisfaction. Based on this framework, the report starts by looking at how key building blocks of Brazil's health system have changed over time and then reviews performance with regard to intermediate and final outcomes. The report is, however, selective, and some important building blocks, such as human resources and pharmaceuticals, are not discussed systematically.

Have the SUS Reforms Transformed the Brazilian Health System?

The SUS reforms envisaged profound changes in the organization and financing of health services as well as the governance and accountability arrangements of the system. Specifically, they targeted several perceived weaknesses of the pre-SUS system, including the limited availability of services in some parts of the country, the weak primary care system, and excessive centralization. The future role of the private sector was debated intensively in the lead-up to the new Constitution; in the end, the Constitution and founding legislation of the SUS defined the role of the private sector as "complementary."

Expansion and Reorganization of Service Delivery

Since the establishment of the SUS, there have been many changes in the organization of service delivery. *Most notably, the capacity of the system has expanded significantly*, with the number of health care facilities growing from nearly 22,000 in 1981 to almost 75,000 in 2009. The growth in facilities was accounted for entirely by expansion of the outpatient network, while the number of hospitals remained fairly stable (from 6,342 to 6,875) and the number of hospital beds actually declined. The expansion of outpatient facilities reflects a growing emphasis on primary care, with the Family Health Strategy (ESF) which was developed based on pilots of integrated primary care in Ceará and other states in the 1980s, being a key driver of this change. Between 1988 and 2010, the number of family health teams increased from 4,000 to more than 31,600, with coverage reaching just over 50 percent of the Brazilian population.

The government's efforts to expand the system were also targeted to addressing regional disparities in access to health services. This is most apparent in the case of hospital beds, where the restructuring of the system significantly reduced the variation in the density of (public) hospital beds across states, and there is now virtually no link between public hospital bed density and average income at the state level. The trend in relation to the distribution of outpatient facilities is less clear. However, the expansion of public outpatient facilities has tended to benefit northeastern states the most. As a result, the density of public facilities is significantly higher in states with low per capita income.

The expansion and restructuring of the delivery network was accompanied by a dramatic decentralization of responsibility for service delivery. The growth in outpatient facilities occurred almost entirely at the municipal level, and the share of hospital beds under municipal control increased from 11 percent to nearly 50 percent between 1985 and 2009. Nonetheless, state and federal levels still manage a significant share of public hospital beds.

The last 20 years also saw a changing mix of public-private hospitals. Although the SUS did not have specific targets for expanding the network of public facilities, policy clearly favored expansion of the public sector over contracting with private providers, reducing both the number of for-profit hospitals under contract and the payment rates to private providers. Reflecting these changes, the share of hospital beds in the public sector increased from 22 to 35 percent, but the private sector still accounts for more than 50 percent of hospital beds.

Toward Increased and More Equitable Health Financing

One of the major accomplishments of the SUS has been *to unify and integrate several independent systems of financing and service provision into a single publicly funded system covering the whole population.*

The SUS reforms also triggered several initiatives aimed at increasing and stabilizing public financing for health, and *government spending on health has increased significantly since the early 1980s*, growing 224 percent in real terms between the first half of the 1980s and 2010 (an 111 percent increase in per capita terms). In part, this growth in government spending on health simply reflects economic growth; while government spending on health as a share of gross domestic product (GDP) fluctuated during the 1980s and 1990s, it has increased significantly since 2003. *Government health spending in Brazil is currently just under 4 percent of GDP, which is significantly lower than the level of spending in most Organisation for Economic Co-operation and Development (OECD) and some middle-income countries*, although Brazil is by no means a clear outlier.

Focusing on the period 1995–2010, for which comparable data from other countries are available, *the average annual rate of growth in (real) per capita government health expenditure was lower in Brazil than in many other middle-income countries* (3 percent a year in Brazil, compared with between 8 and 12 percent in China, the Republic of Korea, South Africa, and Turkey). The growth in real spending picked up in the early 2000s (around 6 percent a year), but it is still lower than in many of Brazil's peers.

Changing Composition of Government Spending on Health

The expansion of the ESF was accompanied by a change in budget allocations, with *federal transfers for "basic care" increasing from 11 to 20 percent of total transfers between 1995 and 2002.* The reallocation of resources in favor of primary care has helped to reduce the hospital-centric nature of the health system, although hospital services continue to account for nearly half of government spending.

Changing Financing Mix across Levels of Government

Reflecting the drastic decentralization of service delivery responsibilities, the financing mix of different levels of government also changed notably over the last two decades. In the late 1980s, immediately after formation of the SUS, federal financing accounted for 85 percent of total government spending on health. Since then, *the federal share of financing has declined steadily, reaching 45 percent in the late 2000s, while municipal and state spending has risen steadily*, reaching 28 and 27 percent, respectively, in 2009.

Shrinking Regional Disparities in Government Spending

While the SUS reforms did not increase government spending on health as much as anticipated, *disparities in government spending across states and municipalities have fallen significantly*. This was achieved not only by making targeted investments in expanding the health system in underserved parts of the country, but also by changing the criteria for allocating federal and state funds for health (Couttolenc 2011b).

The Role of Private Health Financing

When the SUS was established, the importance of the private ("supplemental") health system was expected to decline steadily. This did not happen. Indeed, *despite intentions to the contrary, private spending remained stable over the last 15 years or so* (from around 57 percent of total health spending in 1995 to 54 percent in 2009). *The share of direct out-of-pocket spending declined over time, but still accounts for around 30 percent of total health spending,* while the share of spending on private plans rose and now stands at just over 20 percent. The number of individuals with private health plan coverage grew steadily, but *the share of total health spending financed by government is significantly lower in Brazil than in OECD countries and many middle-income peers.*

Enhancing Health System Governance

For the purposes of this report, governance is seen as being concerned with the management of relationships between various stakeholders in health, including individuals, households, communities, firms, governments of different levels, nongovernmental organizations, private firms, and other entities with the responsibility to finance, monitor, deliver, and use health services. Many of the changes to the health system that the SUS reforms envisaged had important implications for governance and accountability.

One important challenge linked to health system governance is the *establishment and consequences of the right to health*. The right to health was enshrined in the 1988 Constitution and confirmed in the basic legislation of SUS. To operationalize this right, the government expanded the health facility network and maintained the legal provision that anyone can be treated for free under the SUS based on an open-ended benefits package. Inevitably, the SUS has not been able to provide all services for everyone, and many patients have resorted to the courts to seek access to expensive drugs or treatments, resulting in judicial mandates that pose an increasing burden on SUS finances. In recent years, the Ministry of Health has attempted to develop a dialogue with the judiciary and to improve the systems and procedures for incorporating new technologies.

A second important governance challenge concerns the *institutions for coordination and financing across levels of government*. The drastic shift in responsibilities for financing and service delivery to lower levels of government has required new mechanisms for coordination and negotiation across autonomous levels of government. Initially, this effort focused on the establishment of bilateral and trilateral committees. These mechanisms not only improved coordination, but also proved to be bureaucratic and cumbersome. In parallel, new mechanisms for intergovernmental transfers and payments to providers needed to be established, with waves of reforms trying to find a balance between federal direction and local autonomy and between specificity of transfers and the risk of excessive fragmentation. The decentralization process also raised questions about whether some of the 5,600 municipalities that now have primary responsibility for delivering health services are too small to achieve economies of scale and scope in managing the health system. Reflecting this concern, there are ongoing efforts to define a new level of organization of the system—regional health networks—that sits between the state and municipal levels.

A third area related to health system governance concerns *social participation and voice*. Democratization in the health system was a major objective of the SUS reform, and this goal was reflected in the establishment of health councils at each level of government. These councils provide formal mechanisms for society participation, but vary greatly in effectiveness.

Finally, the SUS reforms and subsequent policies have led to changing *purchaser–provider relationships*. In the early 1980s, most payments to private hospitals were done on the basis of fee-for-service, while public providers were financed on the basis of traditional line-item budgets. Over time, fee-for-service payment was replaced by a prospective payment mechanism based on medical procedures (known as the authorization for hospital admission). In parallel to the early rounds of payment reform, several initiatives have sought to develop new organizational models for delivering services. Most prominently, São Paulo pioneered contracting private not-for-profit organizations (*organizações sociais*), and other states and municipalities have followed suit. While the São Paulo model is deemed successful, there is less evidence on performance in other parts of the country. Moreover, limited capacity in contract design and monitoring has often proved to be a significant constraint. Overall, innovations in organizational models, provider payment, and contracting are limited, but gaining momentum (La Forgia and Couttolenc 2008).

Have the SUS Reforms Led to Better Outcomes?

While the SUS reforms focused on transforming how the health system was financed and organized, the ultimate goal was to universalize access to health services. The report assesses the extent to which this goal has been achieved and looks at progress in relation to other intermediate health system goals, in particular quality and efficiency, as well as in relation to the ultimate goals of the health system: improving health outcomes, reducing the financial burden of health expenditures, and enhancing trust and satisfaction with the health system.

Trends in the Use of Health Services

Universality was a key founding principle of the SUS. Universal access or coverage is typically understood to mean that all people have access to a full spectrum of services without suffering financial hardship. Formally, the SUS reforms achieved this goal by decree, but to what extent has this formal entitlement translated into increased access and enhanced financial protection in practice?

SUS "Coverage" and the Persistent Fragmentation of the Health System

In 1981, 49 percent of the population reported that Social Security or the National Institute for Social Medical Assistance (Instituto Nacional de Assistência

Médica da Previdência Social, INAMPS) was their "regular source of care," while another 19 percent reported that they relied on the public system or free philanthropic services. By 2008, only 58 percent of individuals reported being regular users of the SUS. Hence, if measured based on self-reported "regular sources of care," the goal of bringing a larger share of the population into the public health system has not been achieved. However, other evidence suggests that nearly all Brazilians use SUS services at some point, including a recent study indicating that nearly 90 percent of the population uses the SUS exclusively or in combination with the private sector.

Expansion in the Volume of Services Provided by SUS

Another approach to assessing coverage is to look at the volume of services provided by SUS facilities as a measure of realized access. The number of medical consultations per capita increased 70 percent between 1990 and 2009, with the volume of basic care procedures increasing even more rapidly. In contrast, the quantity of hospitalizations provided by the SUS or INAMPS remained stagnant at around 11.5 million. Administrative data on the volume and composition of services are corroborated by survey data, which show that the share of individuals who reported seeking some form of health care in the last two weeks increased nearly 30 percent between 1986 and 2008 (from 11.3 to 14.4 percent). The type of services used by households also changed over time, with preventive visits and dental consultations accounting for a growing share of all visits.

Convergence in Utilization Rates across States and Socioeconomic Groups

By 2009, all states had achieved rates of at least 2.35 consultations per capita per year, with greater increases in utilization in low-income states. Most states experienced reductions in SUS hospital admission rates. Although geographic disparities in utilization declined some, a significant income gradient remains in average utilization rates across states. Moreover, notable disparities persist across income groups, with higher levels of utilization among high-income groups. For instance, household survey data indicate that utilization rates are around 50 percent higher for the top two deciles than for the bottom two.

Are Health Care Needs Being Met?

Trends and patterns in utilization of health services provide a good indication of realized access. However, simple utilization rates do not shed much light on whether individuals are able to access the preventive, diagnostic, and curative services they need in a timely manner, even though this is a critical element in assessing progress toward improving access and achieving universal coverage.

One way to address this question is to look at coverage of health interventions with a clearly defined target group, such as immunizations, antenatal care, and hospital deliveries. On this metric, *Brazil is a stellar performer, with nearly universal coverage and limited geographic disparities.*

Another approach to assessing the extent to which needs are being addressed is to look at self-reported unmet need. *Household surveys found a reduction in unmet need, as well as in the share of households reporting lack of money as a reason for not using services*, in particular for those at the lower end of the income distribution. Meanwhile, facility-related reasons (lack of or unfriendly staff, inadequate scheduling, waiting time) have increased, becoming the chief motive for not seeking care.

Many care-seeking experiences involve multiple providers and services (general practice, specialist care, diagnostic services), with effective access depending not only on the availability of services, but also on the organization and coordination of care, referral arrangements, and other factors. Access is harder to assess in relation to these types of services, but waiting times provide an important metric of unmet need. In this regard, a recent study of cancer care by the Federal Audit Tribunal found that, as a result of weaknesses in primary care and access to diagnostic procedures and specialist care, 60 percent of cancer patients were diagnosed at a very late stage (stage three or four), reducing the prospects of effective treatment and survival. The problem of late diagnosis is compounded by delays in accessing treatment, with median waiting times in 2010 ranging from 76.3 to 113.4 days depending on the type of treatment. The data on diagnosis and treatment delays compare very poorly with available data from OECD countries.

Along similar lines, a study on the demand for specialist, diagnostic, and surgical procedures in Rio Grande do Sul found that, for the state as a whole, with a population of 10.6 million people, there was an unmet need of nearly 500,000 consultations or procedures, mostly in the area of specialist consultation and diagnostic procedures.

The Quality Dimension: A Missing Piece of the Puzzle?

Discussions of coverage tend to focus on access to and cost of services for different groups. However, this concept of "coverage" does not adequately capture quality and the extent to which improvements in coverage of health services translate into better health outcomes. In other words, not only do individuals need to access services, but also those services need to be of appropriate quality and well delivered if potential health gains are to be realized.

Limited data exist on the quality of health care in Brazil, but several studies point to significant concerns with regard to staff training, appropriateness of care, use of quality assurance systems or procedures, and compliance with licensing requirements. There are, however, also signs of improvement, with assessments of quality in the ESF comparing well with the traditional primary care approach and with declines in avoidable admissions.

Health System Efficiency

The concept of efficiency is concerned with the relationship between inputs and outcomes or outputs. At the broadest level, an efficient health system is one that produces the greatest improvement for a given level of spending. However, assessments of efficiency often focus on specific links in the chain from spending to outcomes, including the extent to which resources are allocated appropriately across programs or interventions (allocative efficiency) and the extent to which the greatest volume and quality of health services are produced given available inputs (technical efficiency).

Few studies have looked at *allocative efficiency* in the Brazilian health system, but government spending clearly has been reallocated toward primary care, which is expected to contribute to greater efficiency in the health system.

With regard to the use of *medical technology and allocative efficiency at the facility level*, a substantial proportion of high-complexity equipment is adopted without appropriate consideration of its implications for the cost, quality, and effectiveness of care. Moreover, a substantial proportion of high-cost equipment is installed in municipalities that do not have the size or the role to host it. Notwithstanding partial initiatives in recent years, the Ministry of Health has few established systems for regulating and organizing the adoption and supply of medical technology.

Finally, the report discusses the question of *hospital efficiency*, noting evidence that most Brazilian hospitals operate at a very low level of efficiency. Using data envelopment analysis for a sample of 428 hospitals, the average score for technical efficiency in 2002 was 0.34 on a scale of 0–1. The main factors contributing to inefficiency were small scale of operations, high use of human resources, and low use of installed capacity and technical resources. Indeed, most Brazilian hospitals are too small to operate efficiently, with 65 percent having fewer than 50 beds. Moreover, the mean bed occupancy rate is very low: 37 percent for acute care hospitals and 45 percent for all hospitals.

Improving Health Outcomes: What Has Been the Contribution of the Health System?

Ensuring broad-based access to effective health services was a key concern of the SUS reforms. However, the ultimate goals were to improve the level and distribution of health outcomes, ensure that financing of health care is affordable and equitable, and achieve high levels of responsiveness and satisfaction.

Brazil achieved significant improvements in life expectancy, child and infant mortality, and, to a lesser extent, maternal mortality over the last 20 years. Geographic inequalities in health outcomes were significantly reduced, with northeastern states benefiting the most, and disparities across socioeconomic groups also declined. However, significant inequalities in health status remain.

While the improvements and reduced inequalities in health outcomes are good news, these gains are attributable at least in part to developments outside the health system: access to safe water and sanitation, quality food and education, and the economic situation of households. There is, however, convincing evidence that the SUS has played an important role in improving health outcomes. One approach to assessing the contribution of the health system to better health outcomes is to look at trends in avoidable (or amenable) mortality—that is, deaths that could have been avoided in the presence of timely and effective health care. *Several studies of avoidable mortality in Brazil suggest that SUS has played an important role in improving outcomes, showing that mortality from avoidable causes declined significantly, while mortality from other causes remained stable or even increased.* This result was likely driven at least in part by improvements in coverage and quality of the health system.

In assessing the impact of the health system on health outcomes, evaluations of the ESF provide another piece of the puzzle. *Recent studies have found that implementation of the ESF was associated with significant reductions in infant mortality, diarrhea incidence among children, hospitalization for strokes, and acute respiratory infections in the period between 1990 and 2002.* However, one study reports notable heterogeneity in impact, with large and significant reductions in infant mortality in the North and Northeast and no significant impacts in other parts of the country.

Out-of-Pocket Payments and Financial Protection
The principle of universality is related not only to utilization of services, but also to the extent that individuals are able to access services without financial distress. Improvements in financial protection are typically assessed using data on household spending on health over a defined period. *Available data, which offer data points ranging from 1987 to 2008, suggest that there was little change over time in the share of total household spending dedicated to health,* with estimates ranging from 5 to 7 percent. There was, however, a notable reduction in the share of household spending on health at the lower end of the income distribution in 2002/03 relative to earlier years.

While the overall share of household spending dedicated to health remained stable over the last 20 years, service charges (consultations, hospitalizations, dental care) became relatively less important (declining from 50 percent of out-of-pocket spending in 1987/88 to 20 percent in 2008/09); over the same period, spending on private plans and drugs rose.

The average share of health spending in total consumption provides an important perspective on the burden of health expenditures for households (the incidence of "catastrophic spending"), especially if a large share of it is in the form of out-of-pocket spending. *There is a wide range of estimates for the incidence of catastrophic spending in Brazil. However, the most systematic studies have found low incidence, with Brazil comparing favorably with other countries in the region.* As in many other countries in the region, in Brazil catastrophic spending is significantly higher among poorer households and households with elderly household members (Diniz *et al.* 2007; Knaul *et al.* 2011; Xu *et al.* 2003).

Public Perceptions and Satisfaction with the Health System
The primary goals of the health system are to improve health outcomes and provide effective financial protection. However, most people (and policy makers) also consider satisfaction and responsiveness important intrinsic objectives.

Recent opinion polls concerning the health system in Brazil provide a very mixed picture, reflecting differences in the sample (geographic focus, socioeconomic profile of respondents) and how questions were asked. However, several surveys show high levels of dissatisfaction with public health services, with some surveys suggesting that problems have gotten worse in recent years. The most commonly reported problems are delays in access or treatment and a lack of doctors. However, other surveys provide more positive assessments, with the ESF receiving the most positive assessment.

Of course, given the nearly limitless demand for health care, all countries struggle to meet expectations. Yet dissatisfaction with the health system appears to be particularly high in Brazil. In a recently conducted round of the Gallup World Poll, which asks randomly selected households across a wide range of countries about their satisfaction with public services and other issues, only 40 percent of Brazilians were satisfied with the health system—significantly lower than in many other middle-income countries (such as Malaysia, Thailand, Turkey, or Uruguay) (CNI 2012; Folha de São Paulo 2012; IPEA 2011).

Conclusions

Over the last 20 years, Brazil has seen impressive improvements in health outcomes, with dramatic reductions in child and infant mortality and increases in life expectancy. Equally important, geographic and socioeconomic disparities in outcomes have become far less pronounced. There are good reasons to believe that changes in the SUS have played an important role. The rapid expansion of primary care has contributed to changing patterns of utilization, with a growing share of contacts taking place in health centers and other primary care facilities. There has also been an overall growth in utilization of health services and a reduction in the share of households reporting problems in accessing health care for financial reasons. In short, the SUS reforms have achieved at least partially the goals of universal and equitable access to health care.

This report highlights five primary challenges facing Brazil's health care system in the future.

Sustaining Improvements in Access to Health Care

Progress in this area will depend on sustaining expansion of the ESF. However, it will also be important to recognize the diversity of primary care models that are currently in use and to reach some consensus on their relative merits (and costs). Primary care will also need to be linked effectively with other parts of the health system. Many initiatives are under way to address these challenges: investment and upgrading of capacity, review of payment rates, implementation of clinical guidelines, investment in systems for referrals and electronic medical records, and so forth. In most cases, progress in these areas will require effective coordination across municipalities through regional health care networks. As part of this process, it will also be important to address the lack of integration and clearly define the roles of the public and private sectors. The current lack of coordination between the two sectors results in duplications of efforts and resources, conflicts over who should pay for what, and difficulty addressing systemwide problems.

Improving Efficiency and Quality of Health Care Services

In the face of persistent concerns about efficiency and quality, many states and municipalities are experimenting with new models for providing services, including contracting with nonprofit organizations in Rio de Janeiro, São Paulo, and increasingly in other states. Many parts of Brazil are experimenting with public-private partnerships, in both the construction and management of public facilities. While these contracting arrangements hold promise, they put significant new demands on the state and municipal health secretariats in relation to determining not only what to contract, but also how to design, monitor, and enforce contracts.

New contracting models provide an opportunity to change the way providers are financed and how levels of government coordinate with one another. However, outside of these experiences, weak payment mechanisms contribute to inefficiency and poor quality. Correcting existing distortions and embarking on the large-scale adoption of provider payment methods that provide clear incentives for improving performance would help to make more effective use of available resources and further improve SUS performance within an achievable funding envelope. In the case of public providers, payment reform would have to go hand-in-hand with measures to strengthen the financial and managerial autonomy of hospitals if payment-related incentives are to have an impact on performance.

In the future, it will be important to ensure that efforts to improve quality and efficiency in service delivery are systematically evaluated and that the lessons from these evaluations are shared widely among stakeholders in Brazil.

Clarifying Roles and Relationships across Levels of Government

Decentralization can bring many benefits with regard to increased accountability, tailoring of the system to local needs, coordination with other public services, and so forth. Yet many municipalities lack the scale and technical capacity to manage a health system involving all levels of care and complex supporting services. A well-functioning system will depend on effective coordination and collaboration across municipalities, in particular when it comes to specialist and high-complexity services, referral systems, and medical logistics. It will also depend on robust institutions and approaches for contracting and financing across levels of government. In both of these areas, Brazil has made significant strides in recent years, with new legislation to support a framework for contracting between federal government and health regions and institutional mechanisms for coordinating between municipalities, states, and federal government.

However, implementation of this legislation will inevitably raise many political and practical challenges relating to the process of regional planning, the management and coordination of "shared" services, the financing of investments in systems and capacity to support regional networks, the sharing of financing responsibilities across levels of government, and so forth. States will proceed with this process at different speeds, and it will be important to study and learn from the early adopters.

Raising the Level and Efficiency of Government Spending

There is continuous pressure from the health establishment to increase public funding to health. The report presents data showing that spending increased significantly over the last 20 years in absolute terms (and to a lesser extent as a share of GDP). However, the growth in spending was slower than in many other middle- and high-income countries, particularly in those where coverage expanded rapidly (for example, Korea, South Africa, Thailand, and Turkey). The increase in spending did not keep up with the rapid expansion of the system and the volume of services provided, particularly if cost increases associated with the introduction of new drugs and procedures are considered. More government spending on health would undoubtedly help to finance more health system resources (facilities, equipment, staff), medical supplies, and services.

Yet the report shows that the lack of resources and supplies is in many cases not the binding constraint to improving access and quality. The health system clearly could produce more health services and better health outcomes with the same level of resources if it were more efficient. For instance, significant gains could be achieved by better aligning hospital capacity with need, enhancing the technical efficiency of hospitals, reducing waste and misuse of funds, and so forth. Gains could also be realized through improved prioritization in the allocation of government spending based on more robust processes for introducing and managing the use of existing and new technologies. There are no simple solutions for dealing with these issues, but there is a wealth of international experience on which Brazil could draw. At the same time, even with improvements in efficiency, spending pressures are unlikely to abate in coming decades. As Brazil continues to grow and develop, the combination of unmet needs in both primary and specialist care, the introduction of new technology, growing demands for health care associated with noncommunicable diseases, and the increase in utilization associated with an aging population is likely to put significant pressure on public spending on health. As in other advanced health systems around the world, it will be essential to enhance efficiency and improve prioritization, but it will also be important to prepare for significant and sustained increases in government spending on health and put in place mechanisms for managing the cost pressures already evident in the system.

Conducting More and Better Health System Monitoring and Research

Brazil has a strong tradition of evidence-based policy making in the health sector and a vibrant health research community. The report highlights the need to build on these strengths by improving the information and evidence to support continued health system reform. For instance, although vast amounts of administrative data on health outcomes, service delivery, and financing are publicly available, data suffer from problems related to poor quality, inconsistent definitions, and the structure of data over time and space. This makes benchmarking of health system performance over time, across space, and internationally difficult in some areas.

Data are also lacking on many important dimensions of performance, including waiting times for elective procedures, quality of care for chronic diseases, and survival rates for specific conditions such as cancer or heart attacks. Data on these types of indicators have played a very important role in understanding and addressing health system challenges in OECD countries and will gain importance in Brazil as the country grapples with issues relating to access, quality, and coordination of care.

Beyond the monitoring of health system performance, the report highlights some areas in which in-depth research is warranted, including on the merits of different service delivery models, the impacts of different approaches to improving quality and efficiency, and approaches to reducing out-of-pocket spending on medicines. These are merely some examples of questions that rigorous research and evaluation, based on strong partnerships between policy makers and the research community, can help to answer and, in that way, contribute to making the Brazilian health system more efficient, effective, and equitable.

References

CNI (Confederação Nacional da Indústria). 2012. *Retratos da sociedade brasileira: Saúde pública*. Pesquisa CNI-IBOPE. Brasilia: CNI.

Couttolenc, B. F. 2011a. "Health System Performance and Accountability Assessment in Brazil." Consultant report, World Bank, Washington, DC.

———. 2011b. "Taking Stock of Performance Reforms at the Sub-National Level in Brazil: Recent Performance Gains Achieved in the Health Sector, Hypotheses on Possible Drivers of Good and Bad Performance." Consultant report, World Bank, Washington, DC.

Diniz, B., L. Servo, S. Piola, and M. Eirado. 2007. "Gasto das famílias com saúde no Brasil: Evolução e debate sobre gasto catastrófico." In *Gasto e consumo das famílias brasileiras contemporâneas*, edited by F. Faiger, L. Servo, T. Menezes, and S. Piola, 143–60. Brasilia: Instituto de Pesquisa Econômica Aplicada.

Folha de São Paulo. 2012. "Insatisfação com a saúde sobe 11 pontos em um ano (2012)." *Folha de São Paulo*, January 25.

IPEA (Instituto de Pesquisa Econômica Aplicada). 2011. *Sistema de indicadores de percepção social: Saúde*. Brasilia: IPEA.

Knaul, F., R. Wong, H. Arreola-Ornelas, and O. Mendez. 2011. "Household Catastrophic Health Expenditures: A Comparative Analysis of Twelve Latin American and Caribbean Countries." *Salud Pública Mexicana* 53 (Suppl. 2): S85–95.

La Forgia, G. M., and B. F. Couttolenc. 2008. *Hospital Performance in Brazil: In Search of Excellence*. Washington, DC: World Bank.

Xu, K., D. B. Evans, K. Kawabata, R. Zeramdini, J. Klavus, and C. J. Murray. 2003. "Household Catastrophic Health Expenditure: A Multicountry Analysis." *Lancet* 362 (9378): 111–17.

CHAPTER 1

Introduction

It has been more than 20 years since Brazil's 1988 Constitution formally established the Unified Health System (Sistema Único de Saúde, SUS). Building on reforms that started in the 1980s, the SUS represented a significant break with the past, establishing health care as a fundamental right and duty of the state and initiating a process of fundamentally transforming Brazil's health system to achieve this goal.

As in all health systems, reform begets further reform, such that the process never quite ends. Nonetheless, after 20 years of implementation, it is apt to ask what the SUS has achieved to date and what challenges remain in achieving the goals established in 1988. Such an inquiry is particularly apt now because the demands placed on and the expectations of the health system are growing rapidly. Over the past 20 years, Brazil has experienced profound economic, political, and demographic changes. After considerable turmoil in the 1960s, 1970s, and 1980s, political and economic stability was achieved in the mid-1990s, and economic growth took off in the early 2000s.[1] Economic growth, steadily rising employment, increases in the minimum wage, and social transfer programs all contributed to higher household income and lower poverty and inequality.[2] Recent decades have also seen a profound demographic transition, with a near doubling of the elderly population (60 years of age and older) between 1960 and 2010, from 5.3 to 10.2 percent of the population (World Bank 2011). This economic, social, and demographic transition has had profound implications for the health system, with expanding and changing health needs and rising expectations of what the health system can and should deliver.

This report aims to answer two main questions.[3] First, have the SUS reforms transformed the health system as envisaged 20 years ago? Second, have the reforms led to improvements with regard to access to services, financial protection, and health outcomes?

In addressing these questions, the report revisits ground covered in previous assessments, but also brings to bear additional or more recent data and places Brazil's health system in an international context. The report shows that the health system reforms can be credited with significant achievements.

In particular, the last 20 years have seen an impressive expansion in access to and use of primary care, a profound restructuring of the health system—in particular, a steady decentralization of responsibilities to municipalities—and a rise in government spending on health. There is convincing evidence that some of these reforms have contributed to improvements in health outcomes. Yet, perhaps inevitably, many challenges remain. Access to diagnostic services and specialist care is problematic for large segments of the population; services are fragmented and coordination of care is weak; and service delivery is often poor quality and inefficient in many contexts. As a result of these issues, health outcomes are not as good as they could be, private spending continues to account for a large share of health spending, and levels of satisfaction with the health system are low. There are no silver bullets for addressing these challenges, but the report points to some promising directions for health system reforms that will allow Brazil to continue building on the achievements made to date.

Although it is possible to reach some broad conclusions, there are many gaps and caveats in the story. Given the inherent challenges in assessing health system performance, this is neither surprising nor unusual. Nonetheless, a secondary aim of the report is to consider how some of these gaps can be filled through improved monitoring of health system performance and future research.

The remainder of this introduction presents a short review of the history of the SUS, describes the core principles that underpinned the reform, and offers a brief description of the evaluation framework used in the report. Chapter 2 presents findings on the extent to which the SUS reforms have transformed the health system, focusing on delivery, financing, and governance. Chapter 3 asks whether the reforms have resulted in improved outcomes with regard to access to services, financial protection, quality, health outcomes, and efficiency. The concluding chapter presents the main findings of the study, discusses some policy directions for addressing the current shortcomings, and identifies areas for further research.

SUS: Origins and 20 Years of Implementation

The Brazilian Unified Health System was formally established by the 1988 Constitution, with details outlined in Laws 8.080 and 8.142 of 1990.[4] Prior to establishing the SUS, Social Security institutions—in particular, the National Institute for Social Medical Assistance (Instituto Nacional de Assistência Médica da Previdência Social, INAMPS)—formed the cornerstone of the health system, with the Ministry of Health (Ministério da Saúde) focusing primarily on public health and disease-specific programs. Initially, the Social Security system provided medical coverage only for formal sector workers, primarily through contracts with private sector providers; states and philanthropic organizations provided services for the rest of the population. However, by the late 1970s, rural workers, the self-employed, and domestic workers had been included. INAMPS also provided emergency coverage for the entire population.

The impetus for the SUS came in part from rising costs and a crisis in the Social Security system, but also from a broad-based political movement calling for democratization and improved social rights. In the health sector, the "sanitary movement" (*movimento sanitário*) championed far-reaching health system reforms (Cornwall and Shankland 2008). Protagonists of the movement pointed to chronic underfunding, duplication and inefficiency due to fragmentation and a lack of systemwide coordination, and unequal access to care as key problems of the system. Most important, they argued for a shift away from the "curative privatizing model" that prevailed in the 1970s and early 1980s. This model was premised on the expansion of Social Security coverage to workers outside the original target population, prioritization of curative personal medical care over collective public health programs, the establishment of a "medical-industrial complex," and the migration of service provision to private providers (Silva 1983).[5]

Significant health system reforms were introduced in the 1980s, initially through implementation of "integrated health activities," which sought to improve the coordination among levels of government and reduce duplication in the health system. Later, in the mid-1980s, a second phase of reform turned attention to rearranging institutional roles within the system and decentralizing responsibilities to states and municipalities through establishment of the Unified and Decentralized Health System (SUDS). These reforms, and the Eighth National Health Conference in 1986, laid the foundations for the SUS.

As stated in the Constitution and its basic laws, the SUS has three overarching principles:

- Universal access to health services, with health defined as a citizen's right and an obligation of the state
- Equality of access to health care
- Integrality and continuity of care.

These overarching principles were underpinned by others, including decentralization of most responsibilities to municipalities and joint financing responsibilities; increased community participation; reorganization of the system to enhance integration, improve coordination, and reduce duplication; patient autonomy and right to information; and enhanced effectiveness through the use of epidemiology to define priorities and allocate resources.

Transforming these principles into reality has been an ongoing process ever since the SUS was founded. The first wave of implementation, from 1988 to 1990, focused on establishing the basic legislation and regulations, including the transfer of INAMPS from Social Security to the Ministry of Health,[6] decentralization to the state level, and establishment of mechanisms for social participation. The second wave, from 1991 to 1995, emphasized detailing the norms and rules of the system's organization, financing, and operation, including the "municipalization" of service delivery and the implementation of financial mechanisms for allocating federal funds. A third wave, starting in the mid-1990s, addressed issues in the organization and provision of health care by emphasizing primary care. The fourth and most recent wave of implementation, starting in the mid-2000s, is addressing efficiency and quality issues by reforming governance of the system as well as contracting and payment mechanisms and by establishing regional health care networks.

A Framework for Assessing SUS Performance

The SUS reforms were very ambitious in scope.[7] What have been the results after 20 years? To what extent has the performance of the health system improved? And how does Brazil compare with other countries? Efforts to answer these questions confront a host of challenges that are inherent to any health system assessment. What are the boundaries of the "health system"? What outcomes are important in assessing health system performance? How should outcomes be measured? What importance should be given to different dimensions of performance in assessing the overall system? To what extent can differences across time and space (for example, countries or states) be attributed to reforms or features of the health system?

Various frameworks are available for assessing health system performance (Hurst and Jee-Hughes 2001; OECD 2002; Roberts *et al.* 2003; Smith, Mossialos, and Papanicolas 2008; WHO 2000, 2007). These frameworks differ in important ways, but also share significant commonalities, not only among themselves, but also with frameworks that have been developed and used previously in Brazil to assess health system performance (box 1.1).

In respect for the "boundaries" of the health system, some frameworks take an expansive view, focusing on all activities whose primary intent is to improve or maintain health (for example, WHO 2000, 2007). Based on this approach, public health functions such as disease control, injury prevention, protection against environmental hazards, and food and drug safety should all be considered in assessing the performance of the health system. Other frameworks focus explicitly on the health *care* system and exclude most public health activities and other wider issues (for example, OECD 2002; Hurst and Jee-Hughes 2001). This report largely follows the latter approach: it touches on some issues relating to public health, but is concerned primarily with the financing and delivery of health care.

When it comes to health system goals, there are notable differences in terminology across assessment frameworks, but broad agreement on the ultimate aims of health systems: to improve the level and distribution of health outcomes, responsiveness, and financial protection. In addition to these intrinsic goals, some frameworks also highlight important *intermediate* outcomes, including access and coverage, efficiency, quality, and sometimes others.[8] Finally, many health system performance assessment frameworks identify key health system functions or elements (sometimes referred to as "building blocks" or "control knobs"), which are subject to policy and important determinants of health system performance. The list varies across frameworks, but financing, service delivery, governance, and

Box 1.1 Assessment of Health System Performance in Brazil: Approaches and Recent Developments

The approach adopted in this study is consistent with models and frameworks already developed or adapted in Brazil, including the Ministry of Health's Health Sector Performance Assessment Policy of 2006, the framework of the State Secretariat of Health of São Paulo, the Primary Health Care Assessment Tool of the Ministry of Health, the Quality Improvement Program for Private Health Plans of the National Regulatory Agency for Private Health Insurance and Plans (Agência Nacional de Saúde Suplementar, ANS), and the Programa de Avaliação do Desempenho do Sistema de Saúde (Program for Evaluation of Health System Performance) methodology of the Oswaldo Cruz Foundation (see Couttolenc 2011a) for a review of these models and frameworks).

Recently, the Ministry of Health launched an initiative to monitor the performance of state and municipal health systems. A composite indicator of performance at the municipal level—the SUS Performance Indicator (Índice de Desempenho do SUS, IDSUS)—was developed, based on 24 indicators in five broad areas:

- Access and coverage in basic care (coverage by family health teams, coverage by oral health teams, and percentage of live births from mothers with seven or more antenatal care consultations)
- Access to medium-complexity outpatient and hospital care (coverage of screening for cervical cancer, mammography tests, selected outpatient procedures, and medium-complexity clinical and surgical admissions)
- Access to high-complexity and referral outpatient and inpatient care (coverage of selected high-complexity procedures, high-complexity clinical and surgical admissions, medium- and high-complexity services to nonresidents in the municipality)
- Effectiveness of basic care (percentage of admissions for conditions sensitive to basic care, incidence rate for congenital syphilis, percentage of new cases of tuberculosis and Hansen's disease cured, coverage of dengue tetravalent vaccine, coverage of group-supervised tooth brushing, and proportion of tooth extractions over all dental procedures)
- Effectiveness of medium- and high-complexity care and emergency care (percentage of normal deliveries, intensive care unit mortality among children ages 15 and younger, and mortality from acute myocardial infarction admissions).

The launch of the indicator and the first ranking of states and municipalities have sparked a lively debate. There are legitimate concerns about the choice of indicators, consistency and lags in the data (in some areas, the data refer to 2008 or 2009), the approach to grouping small municipalities, and the weights ascribed to each indicator in constructing the overall index.

Nonetheless, IDSUS represents a big step forward in performance measurement in its clear focus on measuring outcomes rather than processes and commitment to transparency (data are available on the Ministry of Health website). As methodological and data issues are resolved and trend data become available, IDSUS has the potential to become an important tool for monitoring and benchmarking performance across subnational entities.

Figure 1.1 A Simple Framework for Assessing the Performance of the Health System

Health system building blocks	Intermediate outcomes	Final outcomes

• Service delivery and organization
• Financing and resource allocation
• Governance and stewardship
• Human resources
• Information
• Medical products and technologies
	• Access and coverage
	• Quality and safety
	• Efficiency
	  Level and distribution
		• Health outcomes
		• Financial protection
		• Responsiveness and
		  satisfaction
		  Level and distribution

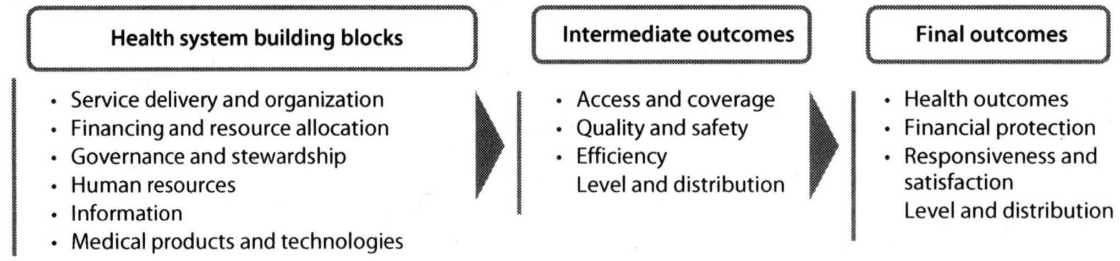

Sources: Based on various health system performance frameworks, including Hurst and Jee-Hughes 2001; OECD 2002; WHO 2000, 2007; Roberts *et al.* 2003; Smith, Mossialos, and Papanicolas 2008.

human resources feature in many of them. Building on the approaches highlighted above, our assessment of the SUS and the structure of this report are based on the simple framework outlined in figure 1.1.

Given the focus on assessing a reform *process* (as opposed to performance of the health system at one point in time), the report starts by looking at how key elements or building blocks of the health system have changed over time. In doing so, the objectives and principles defined by the founding legislation of the SUS provide the starting point. In particular, given the emphasis of the SUS reforms on expanding access, enhancing primary care and health system integration, increasing public spending on health, and achieving decentralization, much of chapter 2 reviews changes in the structure and organization of service delivery, as well as the financing of health services. The report also looks at selected elements of health system governance and accountability. Other health system functions or building blocks—notably human resources, information, and the production and management of medical products and technologies—receive less attention because they featured less prominently in the original SUS vision for reform and because the last two areas (production and management of medical products and technologies) have less impact on the final outcomes of interest in the assessment.

Chapter 3 then reviews performance with regard to intermediate and final outcomes, focusing first on access and coverage, quality, and efficiency and then on the extent to which the health system has improved health outcomes, reduced the financial burden on households, and achieved higher levels of satisfaction.

Performance of the system is assessed with reference to a broad range of indicators relating to inputs, outputs, and outcomes. For most indicators, 1985 (or the closest year) is used as a reference point for comparison over time. As with any assessment of health system performance, this report had to contend with various data limitations, with the most significant challenges being the lack of consistent data over time (due to definitional, measurement, or data quality issues) and the dearth of data for the period before reform. In areas where household or subnational data are available, these are used to shed light on disparities in outcomes.

For the most part, performance is assessed in relation to levels or outcomes before reform and to any goals or targets established at the outset of reform.

Insofar as possible, the report tries to determine the extent to which improvements in outcomes (for example, access, health status, or financial protection) can be attributed to changes in the building blocks or functions (for example, service delivery or financing) of the health system. In some areas, this can be achieved by looking at the relative performance of states or municipalities with different coverage or timing of reforms or by focusing on outcomes that can be linked more directly to changes in the health system. However, neither approach can provide a complete picture. The assessment also puts trends and levels of key indicators in an international context, thereby providing a comparative perspective on performance and remaining challenges.

Contribution of This Report

In recent years, several efforts have been made to assess the SUS reforms and the performance of the Brazilian health system more broadly (for example, Passos 2010; CONASS 2006; Medici 2011; Paim *et al.* 2011; Economist Intelligence Unit 2010; Victora *et al.* 2011; Wagner 2008). Most of these assessments point to a mix of important advances and serious shortcomings.

There is significant agreement on the strengths of the SUS, with improved access and outcomes and successful programs and initiatives in primary health care and public health being the most cited. There is somewhat less agreement on the weaknesses of the system. Some authors emphasize the remaining gaps relative to coverage and access, quality of care, and persistent fragmentation. Others highlight inefficiency, the inability of reforms to confront old vices of the public sector (for example, patrimonialism, capture by health professions and private interests, and weak management), and lack of innovation in the sector. There is, however, broad agreement on the need to improve the performance of the system to meet the expectations and needs of a rapidly aging population, with expansion of primary care, establishment of regional health networks, new models of service delivery (increased autonomy or contracting approaches) for hospitals and primary health care, and quality assurance programs as recurring strategies.

Building on these earlier assessments, this report seeks to provide an objective assessment of the performance of the system and the challenges ahead. The report expands on earlier efforts in several areas, with updated data and more in-depth discussion of government spending on health, intergovernmental finance, and out-of-pocket expenditures. Furthermore, by comparing the achievements of the SUS against three benchmarks—the original objectives of the SUS, the pre-SUS characteristics of the health system, and the achievements of health systems in comparable countries—the report provides a comprehensive discussion of the evolution of the government health system, its successes to date, and remaining challenges.

The report also attempts to reconcile the evidence on expansion in access and use with high levels of public dissatisfaction, pointing to important areas of unmet need and widespread problems with regard to accessing specialist care and many diagnostic services. Finally, the report reviews and summarizes evidence on how health system reforms over the last couple of decades have contributed to improved outcomes. This requires looking beyond high-level trends in mortality and morbidity to take into account recent research on hospital admissions for conditions sensitive to primary care, avoidable mortality, and impact of the expansion of the Family Health Strategy.

Based on this analysis, the report offers recommendations that not only are based on the diagnosis presented and the experiences of other countries in addressing similar reforms but also reflect the operational and political complexities of policy making. It also identifies key gaps in evidence and how additional data and research may be able to shed light on important policy challenges in the health sector.

Notes

1. The average gross domestic product (GDP) growth rate between 2004 and 2010 was approximately 4.4 percent (Ferreira de Souza 2012).

2. The incidence of extreme poverty (US$1.25 purchasing power parity a day) fell from 16.4 to 4.7 percent of the population between 1995 and 2009; inequality, as measured by the Gini coefficient, fell from 0.599 to 0.539 over the same period (Ferreira de Souza 2012).

3. The report is based on three background papers: a review of health system performance and accountability in Brazil (Couttolenc 2011a), an assessment of the Family Health Strategy (Macinko 2011), and a report on equity in the Brazilian health system (Rocha 2011). It also draws from a recent analysis of state-level performance under the SUS (Couttolenc 2011b) and a recent World Bank book on the implications of aging in Brazil (Gragnolati et al. 2011).

4. For a detailed account of the process leading up to establishment of the SUS, see Lima et al. (2005).

5. Private providers under contract with INAMPS constituted the larger part of the INAMPS system, jumping from 26.5 percent of INAMPS total expenditure in 1984 to 55 percent in 1987 (Couttolenc 2011a).

6. INAMPS was formally abolished only in 1993.

7. This section is based on a detailed review of approaches to assessing health system performance that was conducted as a background paper for the study. Counterparts in the Ministry of Health reviewed the framework used in this assessment and found it to be consistent with past and current efforts of the Ministry of Health aimed at evaluating the performance of the Brazilian health system.

8. These are "intermediate" goals in the sense that they are valued not in their own right, but for their contribution to outcomes.

References

CONASS (Conselho Nacional de Secretários de Saúde). 2006. SUS: Avanços e desafios. Brasilia: CONASS.

Cornwall, A., and A. Shankland. 2008. "Engaging Citizens: Lessons from Building Brazil's National Health System." Social Science Medicine 66 (10): 2173–84.

Couttolenc, B. F. 2011a. "Health System Performance and Accountability Assessment in Brazil." Consultant report, World Bank, Washington, DC.

————. 2011b. "Taking Stock of Performance Reforms at the Sub-National Level in Brazil: Recent Performance Gains Achieved in the Health Sector, Hypotheses on Possible Drivers of Good and Bad Performance." Consultant report, World Bank, Washington, DC.

Economist Intelligence Unit. 2010. *Broadening Healthcare Access in Brazil through Innovation*. London.

Ferreira de Souza, P. 2012. "Poverty, Inequality, and Social Policies in Brazil, 1995 to 2009." IPC-IG Working Paper 97, International Policy Centre for Inclusive Growth, Brasilia.

Gragnolati, M., O. Jorgensen, R. Rocha, and A. Fruttero. 2011. *Getting Old in an Older Brazil: Implications of Population Aging on Economic Growth, Poverty Reduction, Public Finance, and Service Delivery*. Directions in Development Series. Washington, DC: World Bank.

Hurst, J., and M. Jee-Hughes. 2001. "Performance Measurement and Performance Management in OECD Health Systems." Labour Market and Social Policy Occasional Paper 47, OECD Publishing, Paris.

Lima, N., S. Gerschman, F. Edler, and J. Suárez, eds. 2005. *Saúde e democracia: História e perspectivas do SUS*. Rio de Janeiro: Editora Fiocruz.

Macinko, J. 2011. *A Preliminary Assessment of the Family Health Strategy (FHS) in Brazil*. Consultant report, World Bank, Washington, DC.

Medici, A. C. 2011. "Propostas para melhorar a cobertura, a eficiência e a qualidade no setor saúde." In *Brasil: A nova agenda social*, edited by E. L. Bacha and S. Schwartzman, 23–93. Rio de Janeiro: LTC.

OECD (Organisation for Economic Co-operation and Development). 2002. *Measuring Up: Improving Health System Performance in OECD Countries*. Paris: OECD.

Paim, J., C. Travassos, C. Almeida, and J. Macinko. 2011. "O sistema de saúde brasileiro: História, avanços e desafios." Série Saúde no Brasil 1, *thelancet.com* (May 9): 11–31.

Passos, R. P., ed. 2010. *Determinação social da saúde e reforma sanitária*. Rio de Janeiro: CEBES.

Roberts, M., W. Hsiao, P. Berman, and M. Reich. 2003. *Getting Health Reform Right: A Guide to Improving Performance and Equity*. New York: Oxford University Press.

Rocha, R. 2011. "Equidade no sistema de saúde brasileiro." Consultant report, World Bank, Washington, DC.

Silva, P. 1983. "O perfil médico-assistencial privatista e suas contradições: A análise política da intervenção estatal em atenção à saúde na década de 70." *Cadernos FUNDAP* 3 (6): 27–50.

Smith, P., E. Mossialos, and I. Papanicolas. 2008. "Performance Measurement for Health System Improvement: Experiences, Challenges, and Prospects." Background document, World Health Organization on behalf of the European Observatory on Health Systems and Policies, Copenhagen.

Victora, C., E. Aquino, M. do Carmo Leal, C. Monteiro, F. Barros, and C. Szwarcwald. 2011. "Saúde de mães e crianças no Brasil: Progressos e desafios." Série Saúde no Brasil 1, *thelancet.com* (May 9): 32–46.

Wagner, G. 2008. "SUS: 20 anos depois." Interview by Cátia Guimarães. Escola Politécnica de Saúde Joaquim Venâncio, Fundação Oswaldo Cruz, Rio de Janeiro, September. http://www.epsjv.fiocruz.br/upload/d/gastao_wagner.pdf.

WHO (World Health Organization). 2000. *World Health Report 2000: Health Systems; Improving Performance.* Geneva: WHO.

————. 2007. *Everybody's Business: Strengthening Health Systems to Improve Health Outcomes; WHO's Framework for Action.* Geneva: WHO.

World Bank. 2011. *World Development Indicators.* Washington, DC: World Bank.

CHAPTER 2

Have the SUS Reforms Transformed the Brazilian Health System?

The reforms of Brazil's Unified Health System (Sistema Único de Saúde, SUS) envisaged a fundamental transformation, with universality, equity, integration, decentralization, and participation as key principles. Needless to say, turning these principles into reality required profound changes to how the health system is financed and organized.

This chapter reviews the evidence on whether and to what extent this transformation has happened, focusing on the expansion and reorganization of service delivery, financing of health services, and governance and accountability arrangements of the system. It finds that significant progress has been made. The capacity to deliver services has expanded, regional disparities in the availability of services have been reduced, primary health care has been strengthened, most of the responsibilities for delivering services have been decentralized to municipalities, government health expenditures have increased, and various institutional mechanisms and innovations have been introduced to enhance coordination, participation, and efficiency. But the chapter also finds that the SUS reforms are an unfinished agenda, with intergovernmental finance and coordination and the evaluation and consolidation of models for contracting, integrating, and delivering health services standing out as important challenges for the future.

Expansion and Reorganization of Service Delivery

Universalization of access to health services and improvements in equity depend critically on the availability of services. In this regard, the SUS reforms targeted several perceived weaknesses of the pre-SUS system, including scarce services in some parts of the country, a weak primary care system, and excessive centralization. While the Eighth National Health Conference (1986) debated gradual nationalization (*estatização*) as a guiding principle of health system reform, the Constitution and subsequent legislation (Laws 8.080 and 8.142) merely defined the national system under construction as public and publicly financed and the private sector's role as "complementary."[1]

Expansion of the Delivery Network and Increased Focus on Primary Care

Since the early 1980s, the Brazilian network of health facilities has expanded significantly, with the number of health care facilities growing from nearly 22,000 in 1981 to almost 75,000 in 2009. This growth in facilities began during the 1970s and 1980s, when the military government promoted expansion of the system through contracts with private providers. However, the SUS reforms signaled an important shift in policy direction and resource allocation, with outpatient facilities accounting for most of the growth in facilities. Indeed, the growth in facilities was accounted for entirely by expansion of the outpatient network, while the number of hospitals remained stable (from 6,342 to 6,875) and the number of hospital beds declined (figure 2.1).

Focusing on the density of facilities and beds, both the number of hospitals and the number of hospital beds per 10,000 population declined over the last 20 years, while the density of outpatient facilities increased almost threefold, from 1.3 facilities per 10,000 population in 1981 to 3.6 in 2009 (figure 2.2).

The growth in outpatient facilities indicates the growing emphasis on primary care over the last couple of decades. A key driver of this change has been the rapid deployment of the Family Health Strategy (ESF) and its sibling, the Community Health Agents Program (PACS).[2] The ESF was piloted in the 1980s in Ceará and some other states and was adopted in 1994 as a national strategy for reorganizing health care delivery in the public system (see box 2.1 for a summary of features of the ESF).[3] The ESF, which forms an integral part of the SUS, was intended to improve the country's existing primary health care services (delivered through basic care units or *unidades de atendimento basico*). Problems with the earlier model included inadequate availability of basic care units, poor geographic distribution, lack of trained health providers (especially physicians), little or no community engagement, widespread dissatisfaction with the quality of services, and

Figure 2.1 Network of Health Facilities in Brazil, 1981–2009

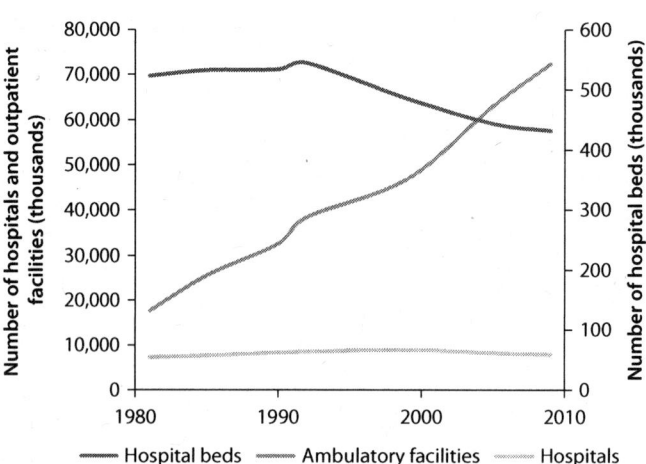

Sources: Data from *Pesquisa de AMS (IBGE, 2010;* IBGE 2010.

Figure 2.2 Density of the Network of Health Facilities in Brazil, 1981–2009

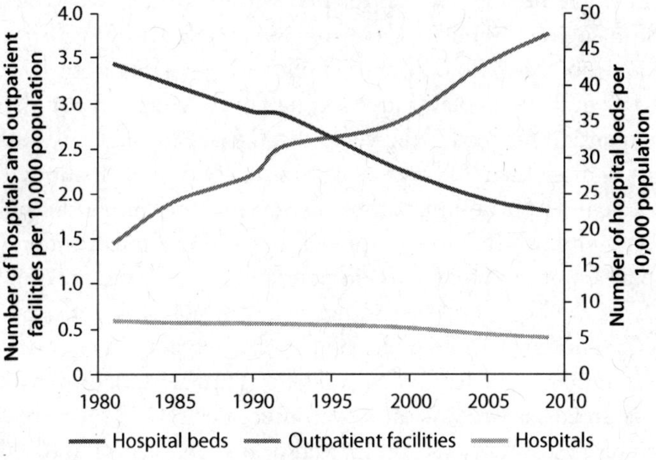

Sources: Data from *Pesquisa de AMS (IBGE, 2010);* IBGE 2010.

Box 2.1 Primary Care and Prevention in Brazil: The Family Health Strategy

The Family Health Strategy was inspired by the Community Health Agents Program, a community health initiative piloted in rural areas of Ceará during the 1980s. The Family Health Strategy (ESF) was initially developed in parallel with the PACS (Programa de Agentes Comunitários de Saúde), gradually replacing it. It was designed to provide first contact, comprehensive, and whole person care coordinated with other health services, emphasizing care that takes place within the context of family and community. In the ESF, multiprofessional health teams (composed of a physician, a nurse, a nurse assistant, and four to six community health workers) are organized by geographic regions, with each team providing primary care to approximately 1,000 families (or about 3,500 people). In 2004, oral health teams were added to the program, filling a long-standing gap in the public system.

The ESF teams are based in basic care units and backed by professionals that are not part of the team. Their activity is heavily focused on prevention and promotion outreach activities, with monthly visits to enrolled families. The ESF was meant to correct the limitations of the facility-centered, passive, and curative approach to care. It includes not only typical primary health care activities, mostly targeting children and women, but also activities focusing on the control of communicable and chronic diseases, including tuberculosis, Hansen's disease, hypertension, and diabetes.

The program is monitored through an intergovernmental "Agreement on Basic Care" (*Pacto de Atenção Básica*) and more recently through a broader "Agreement for Life" (*Pacto pela Vida*), which covers 12 indicators related to the ESF strategy. However, the quality and reliability of the indicators reported are questionable and vary by state.

Sources: Macinko 2011; Schmidt *et al.* 2011; Ministry of Health website.

---

long waiting times. In contrast, the ESF sought to provide first contact, comprehensive, and whole person care coordinated with other health services.[4]

The ESF has grown rapidly: between 1998 and 2010, ESF teams increased from 4,000 to more than 31,600, and enrollment expanded from 10.6 million to more than 100 million people, or just over half of the Brazilian population (figure 2.3). The expansion proceeded unevenly throughout the country, but the ESF is now present in more than 90 percent of Brazil's 5,565 municipalities. The expansion of the ESF has been complemented by several other important public health programs and initiatives focused on prevention and health education (box 2.2).

The expansion of the ESF started in poor and underserved areas of northeastern states. This can be seen clearly in figure 2.4, which shows program coverage by level of economic development of the municipality. After controlling for several confounding variables, Rocha and Soares (2009) found that adoption has tended to be greater in areas with poorer initial health and fewer resources (for example, water and sanitation) and limited or no prior access to health services.

This pattern is also reflected in household survey data. Figure 2.5, using individual-level data from the 2008 *Pesquisa Nacional por Amostra de Domicilios* (PNAD), shows that people listed as enrolled in the ESF are most likely to be found in the lowest-income quintiles and that the proportion of families enrolled in the ESF declines as family income increases (IBGE 2008). Nevertheless, even in the second-richest quintile (quintile 4), more families were covered by the ESF in 2008 than were enrolled in private health insurance plans.

However, after the initial deployment and rapid expansion of the program until around 2002, growth has been slow and uneven (Macinko 2011; table 2.1). Expansion of the program slowed down not only in the early adopters, but also

Figure 2.3 Coverage of the ESF in Brazil, 1994–2010

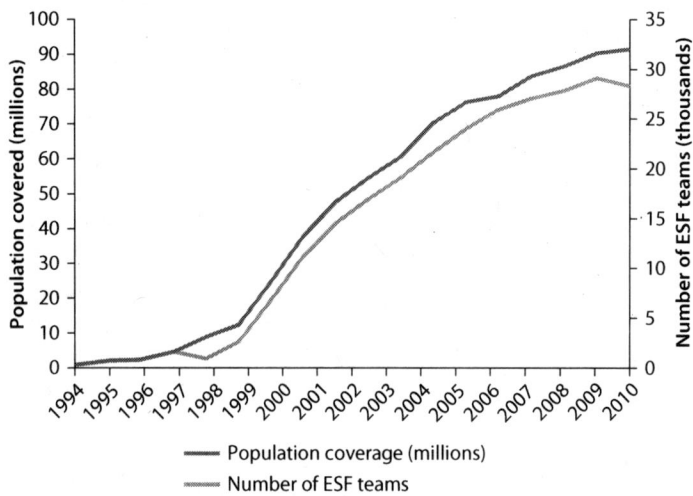

— Population coverage (millions)
— Number of ESF teams

Source: Ministry of Health, DAB 2011.
Note: ESF = Family Health Strategy. Coverage is estimated based on the approach of the Ministry of Health, which entails multiplying the number of teams by 3,450.

Box 2.2 Primary Care and Prevention in Brazil: Beyond the Family Health Strategy

Several new public health programs have been adopted in recent years, testifying to the renewed emphasis on primary care, prevention, and health promotion. The Smiling Brazil Program has expanded access to dental care, and the Popular Drugstores Program has facilitated access to free or subsidized essential drugs, addressing two of the greatest weaknesses in SUS (Sistema Único de Saúde) coverage. Other initiatives have focused on the prevention and control of chronic diseases. The National Tobacco Control Program has changed smoking habits to some extent, and smoking is now prohibited in public places; based on a strong component of health information and education, the program has contributed to the decline in noncommunicable diseases and significantly reduced both the number of tobacco users (from 35 percent of the adult population in 1989 to 16 percent in 2006) and the intensity of use (Iglesias *et al*. 2007).

Other programs focus on the prevention and control of chronic diseases. A program for the control of hypertension and diabetes focuses on routine measurement of blood pressure, pharmaceutical control through the distribution of drugs, and the promotion of exercise. The national programs for the control of breast and cervical cancer focus on prevention, early detection, and treatment of the disease. Psycho-Social Care Centers have been implemented in many municipalities to expand coverage of outpatient mental health services and facilitate the return home of people with mental disorders, and the Program on Alcohol and Drug Abuse aims to reduce the rate of hospitalization for these disorders. These programs are evidence of an increased focus on managing chronic diseases and controlling their risk factors.

More recently, these initiatives were consolidated into one National Plan for the Control of Chronic Non-Transmissible Diseases, which includes (a) surveillance, information generation, research, and monitoring and evaluation; (b) health promotion through a multisectoral approach to addressing risk factors, the promotion and facilitation of exercise and healthy eating, the promotion of active aging, and campaigns to reduce the consumption of tobacco and alcohol; and (c) integral care including screening, early detection, clinical guidelines, free drugs, and emergency and home care.

Sources: Macinko 2011; Schmidt *et al*. 2011; Ministry of Health website.

---

in all groups of municipalities. As a result, larger municipalities (state capitals and metropolitan areas), which were late adopters of the strategy, continue to lag, with coverage rates in the range of 35–45 percent of the population.[5] One possible reason for the stagnation in coverage is the reliance on short-term contracts in many municipalities.[6] These unstable arrangements have been increasingly criticized and challenged on regulatory grounds, which may have prevented municipalities from expanding the program further. However, restrictions on the hiring of civil servants (associated with the Fiscal Responsibility Law, which limits the proportion of the budget that can be spent on personnel) offered little alternative to the outsourcing strategy. Moreover, as Rocha and Soares (2009) found, the probability and timing of a given municipality adopting the ESF was influenced by political factors, with municipalities governed by left-wing parties

Figure 2.4 Coverage of the ESF in Municipalities in Brazil, by Income Quintile, 1985–2007

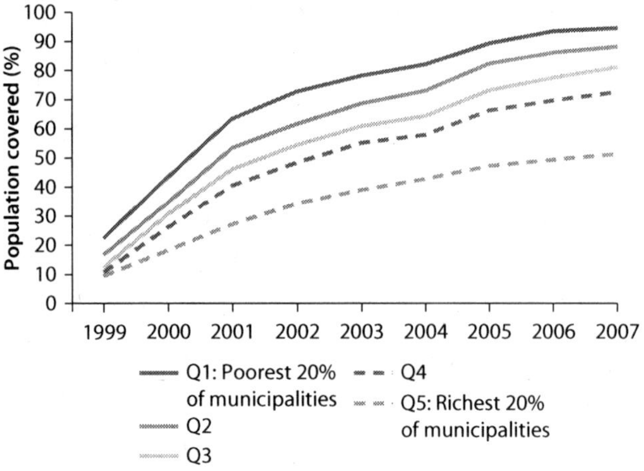

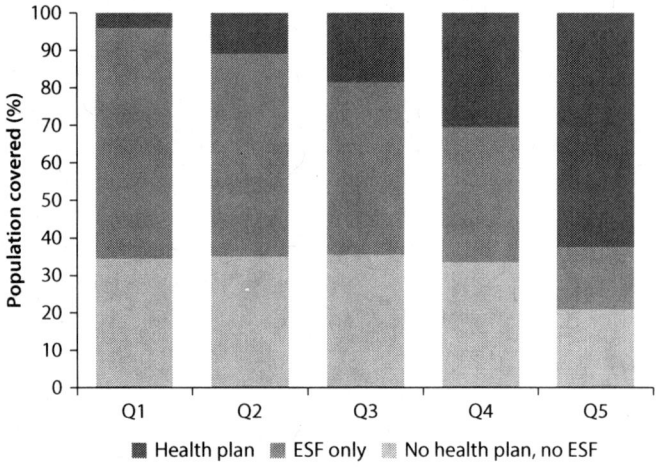

Source: Macinko 2011, from Ministry of Health, DATASUS data.
Note: ESF = Family Health Strategy.

Figure 2.5 Coverage of the ESF in Brazil, by Income Quintile, 2008

Source: IBGE 2008.
Note: ESF = Family Health Strategy. Includes poststratification weights and controls for complex survey design (Macinko 2011).

and by the Brazilian Social Democracy Party (which held power at the federal level from 1994 through 2002) being more likely to adopt it.

As a result of this pattern of expansion, ESF coverage varies significantly, with coverage tending to be higher in the states with low household income per capita (figure 2.6).

In addition to the rapid expansion of outpatient care facilities and the ESF in previously underserved areas, other initiatives have also sought to improve access to specific services, in particular dental care and free medications. These initiatives have targeted states in the Northeast and North, along with other

Table 2.1 Coverage of the ESF and the PACS in Brazil, by Size of Municipality, 1998–2010

Size of municipality	Coverage (% of population)				Change in coverage (%)		
	1998	2002	2006	2010	1998–02	2002–06	2006–10
More than 1 million	2.0	21.0	32.9	36.8	19.0	11.9	3.9
350,000–999,999	4.4	30.5	42.5	45.4	26.1	12.0	2.8
100,000–349,999	9.2	38.4	49.6	56.7	29.2	11.3	7.1
50,000–99,999	17.3	54.5	66.6	71.7	37.1	12.1	5.2
20,000–49,999	20.6	62.7	75.3	87.2	42.0	12.7	11.9
Less than 20,000	23.3	73.8	85.4	98.5	50.5	11.6	13.1

Source: Ministry of Health, Primary Care Information System online database.
Note: ESF = Family Health Strategy, PACS = Programa de Agentes Comunitários de Saúde.

Figure 2.6 Coverage of the ESF in Brazil, by State, 2008

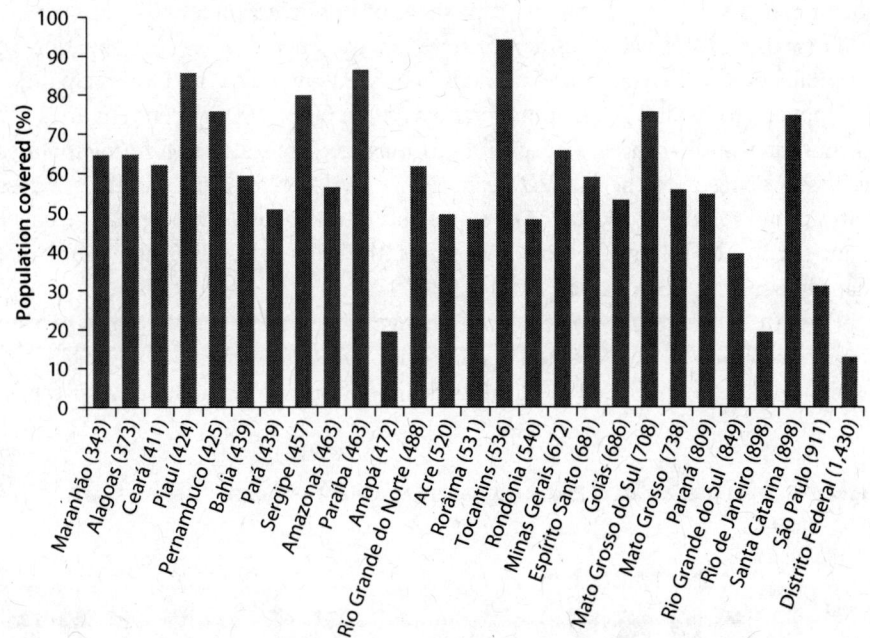

Source: Ministry of Health, DATASUS data.
Note: ESF = Family Health Strategy. States are sorted by household income per capita (in parentheses) IPEA data of the Institute of Applied Economic Research (Instituto de Pesquisa Econômica Aplicada, IPEA).

states with poor indicators (Distrito Federal, Mato Grosso do Sul, Paraná, Rio de Janeiro, and Rondônia).

Of course, in many parts of the country, the traditional model of providing primary care through basic care units is still being implemented, making it difficult to determine coverage of primary health care (as opposed specifically to the ESF). For instance, in Rio de Janeiro Municipality, 599 family health teams were operating from family clinics and health centers in February 2012. This translates into ESF coverage of approximately 33 percent. However, the municipality estimates that an additional 17 percent of the population have access to municipal health centers that offer a more limited package of services and another 30–40 percent of the population have private health plans that cover primary health care.

Decentralization and a Changing Public-Private Mix

The expansion and restructuring of the delivery network were accompanied by a dramatic decentralization of responsibility for service delivery. Indeed, the growth in outpatient facilities occurred almost entirely at the municipal level, and by 2009 virtually no outpatient facilities were under state or federal management (figure 2.7). Decentralization of hospital care has not been as dramatic: the share of hospital beds under municipal control increased from 11 percent to nearly 50 percent between 1985 and 2009, but state and federal governments still manage a significant share of public hospital beds.

There is notable variation across states in the degree of decentralization of hospital beds, with the share of beds managed by states and municipalities (as opposed to federal government) ranging from 60 to 100 percent (figure 2.8). In most states, the share of hospital beds managed by states and municipalities has been rising over the last 20 years. There is also significant variation across states in the relative importance of states and municipalities in hospital management (figure 2.9). However, in most states, the share of beds under municipal management has been rising.

The last 20 years have also seen a change in the mix of public and private service provision in the hospital sector. Prior to establishment of the SUS, the National Institute for Social Medical Assistance (Instituto Nacional de Assistência

Figure 2.7 Decentralization of Public Outpatient Facilities and Hospital Beds in Brazil, 1981–2009

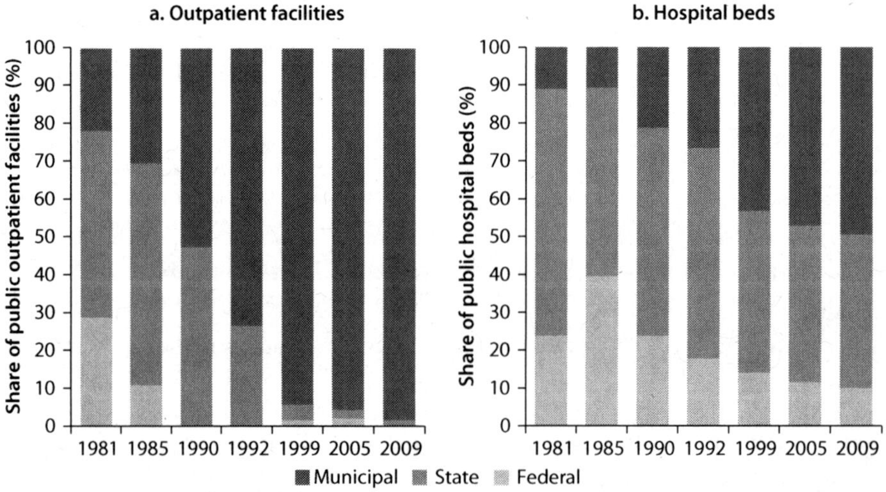

Sources: Data from *Pesquisa de AMS*; IBGE 2010.

Figure 2.8 Local (State and Municipal) Management of Hospital Beds in Brazil, 1992–2009

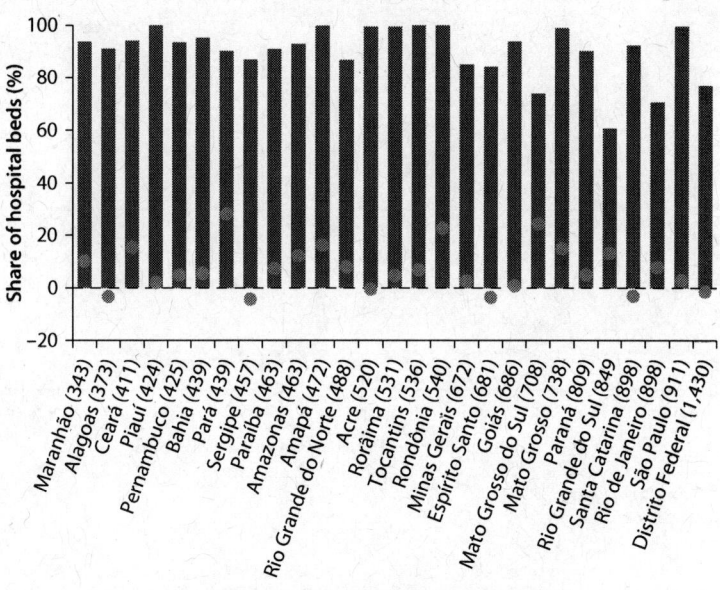

State (household income per capita, R$)

■ Local share (2009)   ● Change in local share, 1992–2009 (% points)

Source: Based on Ministry of Health, DATASUS data.

Figure 2.9 Municipal Management of Hospital Beds in Brazil, 1992–2009

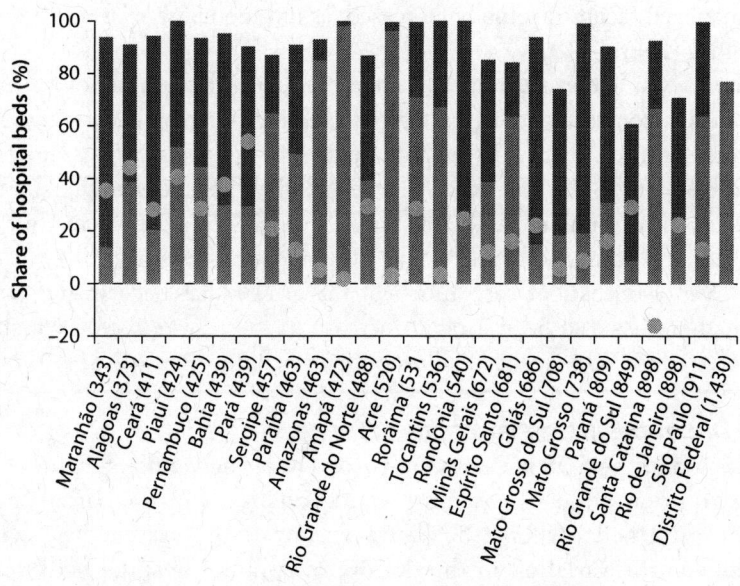

State (household income per capita, R$)

■ Municipal share   ▨ State share   ● Change in municipal share 1992–2009 (% points)

Source: Based on Ministry of Health, DATASUS data.

Figure 2.10 Public-Private Composition of Hospitals and Hospital Beds in Brazil, 1980–2010

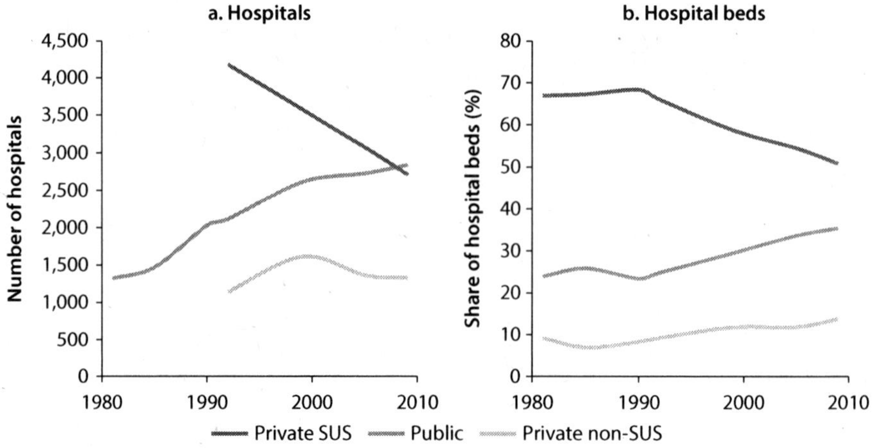

Sources: Data from *Pesquisa de AMS*; IBGE 2010.
Note: SUS = Sistema Único de Saúde.

Médica da Previdência Social, INAMPS) had contracted most hospital care from the private sector. As noted, the SUS did not have specific targets for expanding the network of public facilities, but policy clearly favored expansion of the public sector over contracting with private providers. This is reflected in the data, which show that the slight reduction in the number of hospitals is mainly accounted for by the closure of private hospitals under contract with the SUS (and with INAMPS before the SUS), especially in the for-profit sector. The number of publicly managed facilities actually increased, as did the number of private non-SUS hospitals (figure 2.10).

This change was achieved in part by simply reducing the number of for-profit hospitals under contract and in part by decreasing—in real terms—the SUS payment rates to private providers, which made it impossible for many hospitals to survive based on SUS contracts. As a result of these changes, the share of hospital beds in the public sector increased from 22 to 35 percent, but the private sector still accounts for more than 50 percent of hospital beds.

In the case of outpatient care, much of the growth has been in the public sector, but there has also been a rapid increase in the private sector, which by 2009 accounted for 30 percent of all outpatient facilities (figure 2.11).

Regional Disparities in the Availability of Services
The expansion of the SUS network has helped to reduce regional inequalities in the distribution of health system resources. This is most apparent in the case of hospital beds, where the restructuring of the system has significantly reduced the variation in the density of (public) hospital beds across states (figure 2.12). The trend in relation to the distribution of outpatient facilities is less clear. However, the expansion of public outpatient facilities has tended to benefit northeastern states the most. As a result,

Figure 2.11 Public-Private Composition of Outpatient Facilities in Brazil, 1980–2010

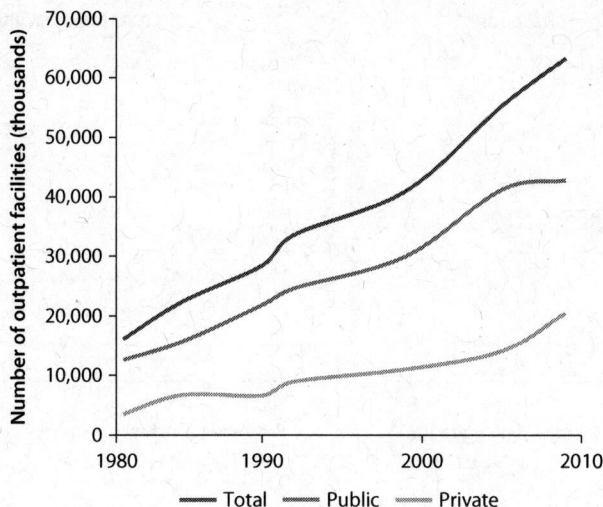

Sources: Data from *Pesquisa de AMS*; IBGE 2010.

Figure 2.12 Density of Hospital Beds and Outpatient Facilities across States in Brazil, 1988 and 2009

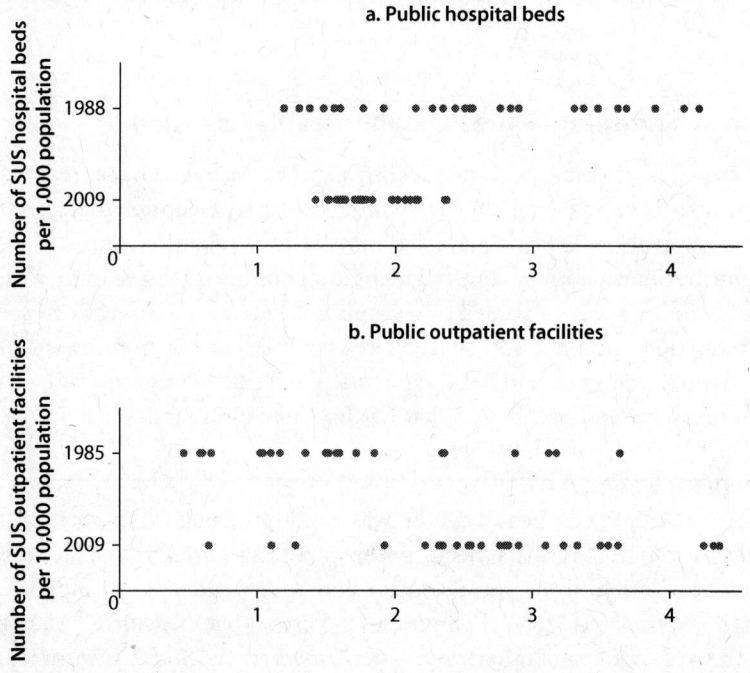

Source: Based on Ministry of Health, DATASUS data.
Note: SUS = Sistema Único de Saúde.

Figure 2.13 Link between Income and Density of Facilities across States in Brazil, 1988 and 2009

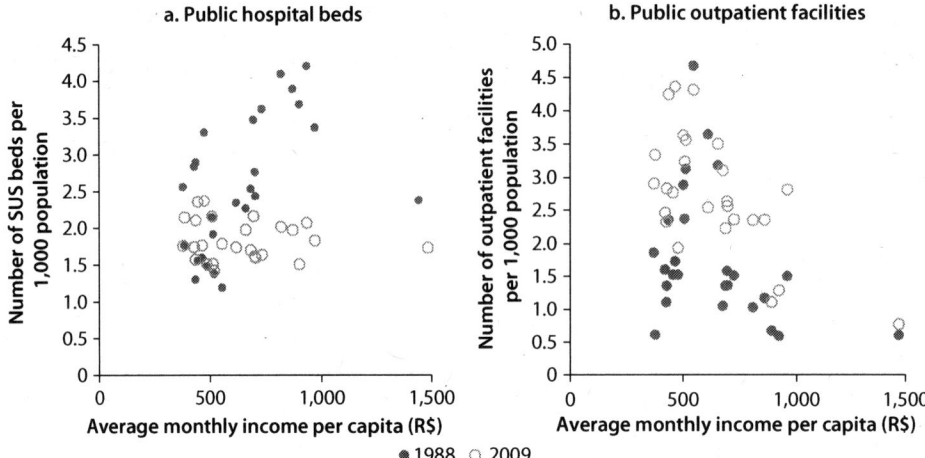

Sources: Based on Ministry of Health, DATASUS data. Data on average monthly income from the Institute of Applied Economic Research (Instituto de Pesquisa Econômica Aplicada, IPEA).
Note: SUS = Sistema Único de Saúde.

the density of public facilities is now significantly higher in states with low per capita income (figure 2.13). The opposite used to be true for public hospital beds, but two decades of restructuring of the public system has delinked the density of public hospital beds from average income at the state level.

Toward Increased and More Equitable Health Financing

While the SUS reforms did not establish explicit goals or targets regarding the sources and mix of financing, they were premised on a perception that government spending on health was inadequate and that the high reliance on private spending was contributing to both system fragmentation and inequalities. Implementation was expected to be accompanied by a significant increase in government spending and a reduction in private spending. Moreover, the reorientation toward primary care and the decentralization were expected to have large impacts on the patterns of both financing and spending. What has happened in practice?

Government Financing

In the early 1980s, the health sector was funded through four main financing schemes or sources: (a) Social Security through the INAMPS, which covered the working population in the formal sector and its dependents; (b) independently managed federal and state government facilities that provided basic services mostly to the poor and other groups not covered by Social Security; (c) the private health insurance system; and (d) direct out-of-pocket payments for drugs and services (mainly provided by the private sector). In other words, the health system was composed of several vertical, independent, and uncoordinated systems;

each had its own source of funding and its own network of facilities and covered a defined population (even when this was simply "population groups not covered by other schemes").

One of the major impacts of the SUS has been to unify and integrate these independent financing and service provision systems into a single publicly funded system covering the whole population.[7] Given the SUS architecture and the shared responsibilities across government levels, financial mechanisms have always been at the core of SUS legislation, regulations, and policies and a major force in organizing the system. As indicated earlier, the first years of SUS implementation focused mostly on designing mechanisms for transferring federal funds to states and municipalities and defining prerequisites for these to receive the transfers. This bureaucratic approach had its downsides (for example, the complex set of administrative regulations and requirements and financial flows), but helped to build the basic architecture and principles that make up the SUS today: financing mechanisms, monitoring and evaluation systems, and negotiating bodies (health councils and committees) that determine resource allocation and set priorities.

Critical elements of the SUS are the health funds established at each level of the system under a single command. Federal taxes and social contributions finance the federal health fund, which in turn finances nearly all Ministry of Health facilities and programs and contributes significantly to the financing of university hospitals (within the Ministry of Education). The federal health fund is a major contributor to state and municipal funds, which are also financed by state and municipal revenues. These federal transfers are a key element of the system, since they are the main incentive for subnational governments to buy into national health policies and priorities and to implement them within a federalist political system.

In principle, municipal governments should, through their municipal health funds, be the main provider and purchaser of health services. However, because most municipalities are small and have limited technical or financial capacity, many facilities and a large part of SUS finance remain at the hands of regional and central authorities.

The SUS reforms also triggered several initiatives aimed at increasing and stabilizing public financing for health. The first, during the late 1980s, sought to earmark a fixed share (30 percent) of Social Security revenues for health. This law was never passed; in fact, at the turn of the decade, health spending was taken out of Social Security altogether and was funded by general revenues and new "social contributions." In the 1990s, a second initiative established a new excise tax earmarked for health (Contribuição Provisória sobre Movimentações Financeiras, CPMF). However, CPMF revenue was never fully allocated to health, and other sources of finance were reduced, such that funds from the CPMF had little impact. Finally, a constitutional amendment passed in 2000 (Constitutional Amendment no. 29) sought to establish a minimum level of government health spending (as a share of overall government spending). It succeeded in increasing state and municipal expenditures by mandating that a minimum share of the budget be allocated to health (12 and 15 percent, respectively), but a corresponding mandate was never approved for the federal budget.

The available evidence indicates that public spending on health has increased significantly since the early 1980s (figures 2.14 and 2.15), growing 224 percent in real terms between the first half of the 1980s and 2010, or from R$339 to R$714 per capita (111 percent growth).[8] Despite this increase in spending over time, expenditures have fluctuated significantly, with a few distinct phases: (a) the first half of the 1980s, when spending oscillated with economic crisis and recovery (which is why the mean value for 1980–85 is used here as the base for comparison); (b) the second half of the 1980s, when expenditure nearly doubled to reach a peak in 1989; (c) a severe drop in 1990–94; (d) stagnation at a higher level from 1995 through 2003; and (e) a period of steady growth starting in 2003, during which expenditure nearly doubled, helped by strong economic growth.

While spending has increased substantially in absolute and per capita terms, the share of government health spending in gross domestic product (GDP) has grown more slowly (figure 2.16). From a level of around 2.5 percent in the early 1980s, it increased rapidly to 4 percent by 1989. In the decades that followed, it oscillated at lower levels, regaining its 1989 level only in 2009. In other words, the initial effort to expand public spending in the late 1980s was not sustained, and spending did not begin to increase notably until 2003. Figure 2.16 also illustrates the strong link between government health spending and the economic cycle: increases during economic expansion and sharp reductions during economic downturns. This link with the economic cycle was a typical feature of public financing before the SUS reforms and has remained in spite of being one of the key concerns of the health reform.

Focusing on the period 1995–2010, for which comparable data from other countries are available, the average annual growth of (real) government health spending per capita was lower in Brazil than in many other middle-income countries (figure 2.17). For instance, while China, the Republic of Korea, South Africa, and Turkey experienced annual rates of growth between 8 and 12 percent, government health spending per capita in Brazil grew at around 3 percent. Government health spending per capita has grown more rapidly since the early 2000s (around 6 percent a year), but is still lower than in many of Brazil's peers.

While growth in spending has been relatively slow, Brazil started from a higher base than many of its peers. Consequently, government spending on health as a share of GDP, currently just under 4 percent, is significantly lower than the level of spending in most Organisation for Economic Co-operation and Development (OECD) countries and some middle-income peers, but Brazil is by no means a clear outlier (figure 2.18). Nonetheless, the slow growth in government spending stands in stark contrast to the rapid expansion of service delivery capacity and volume of services provided through the SUS.

Figure 2.14 SUS and Social Security Spending on Health in Brazil, by Level of Government, 1980–2009

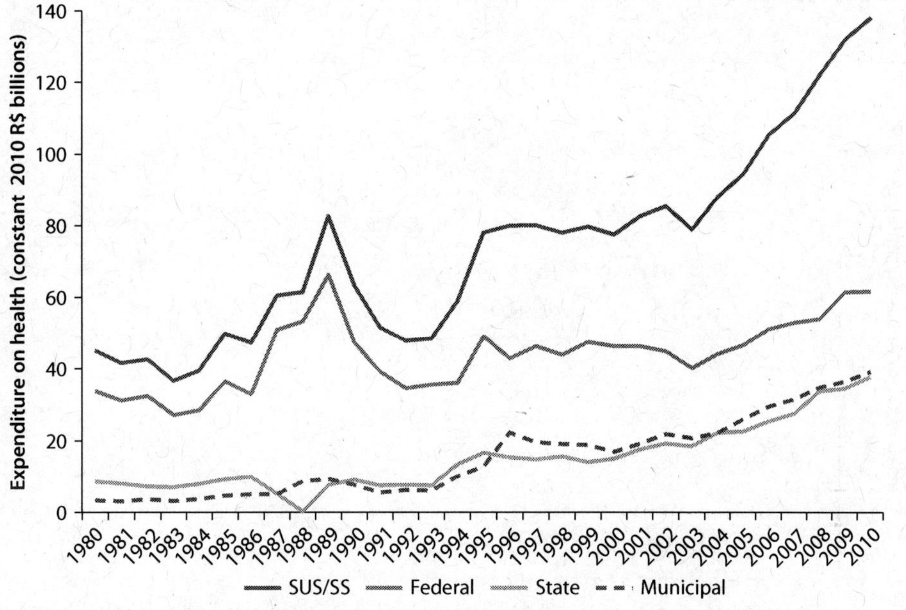

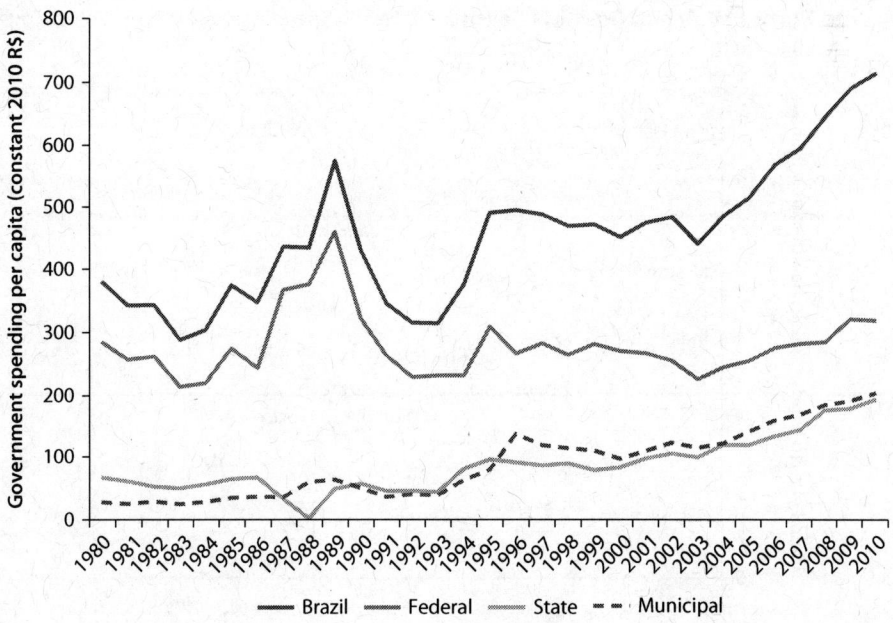

Sources: Based on Ministry of Health, Public Health Budget Information System (SIOPS) data; Ministry of Finance, STN 2010; Medici 1991.
Note: SUS (Sistema Único de Saúde) expenditure includes funding from federal, state, and municipal governments; Social Security (SS) through 1990 includes only federal funding (a mix of payroll contributions and other "social contributions" and taxes).

Figure 2.15 SUS and Social Security Spending per Capita on Health in Brazil, by Level of Government, 1980–2010

Sources: Based on Ministry of Health, SIOPS data; Ministry of Finance, STN 2010; Medici 1991.
Note: SUS = Sistema Único de Saúde.

Figure 2.16 SUS and Social Security Spending on Health as a Percentage of GDP in Brazil, by Level of Government, 1980–2009

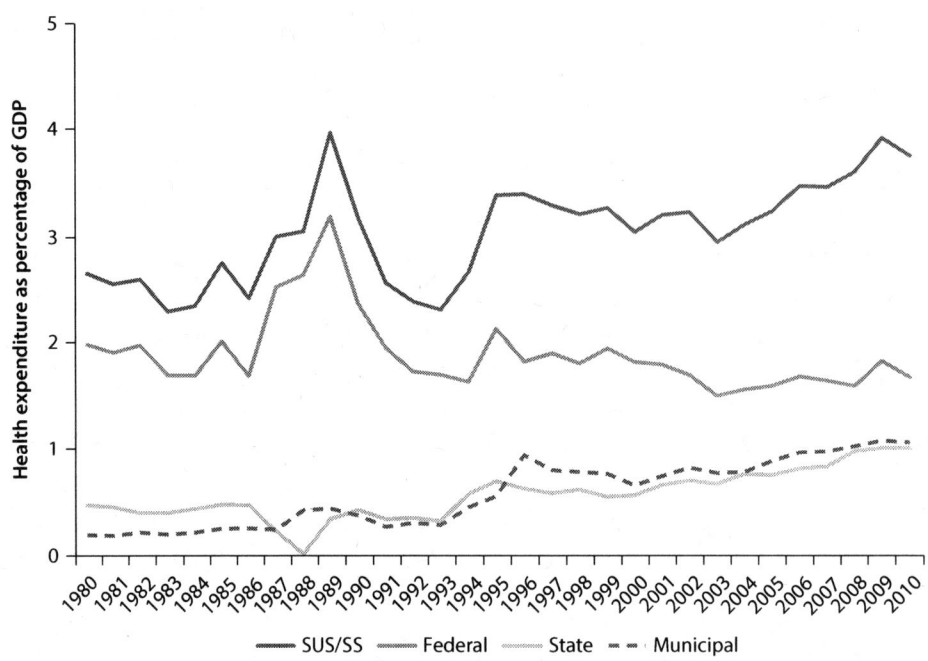

Sources: Based on Ministry of Health, SIOPS data; Ministry of Finance, STN 2010; Medici 1991; IBGE 2010 (for GDP data).
Note: GDP = gross domestic product, SS = Social Security, SUS = Sistema Único de Saúde.

Figure 2.17 Annual Growth in Government Health Spending per Capita in Select Countries, 1995–2010

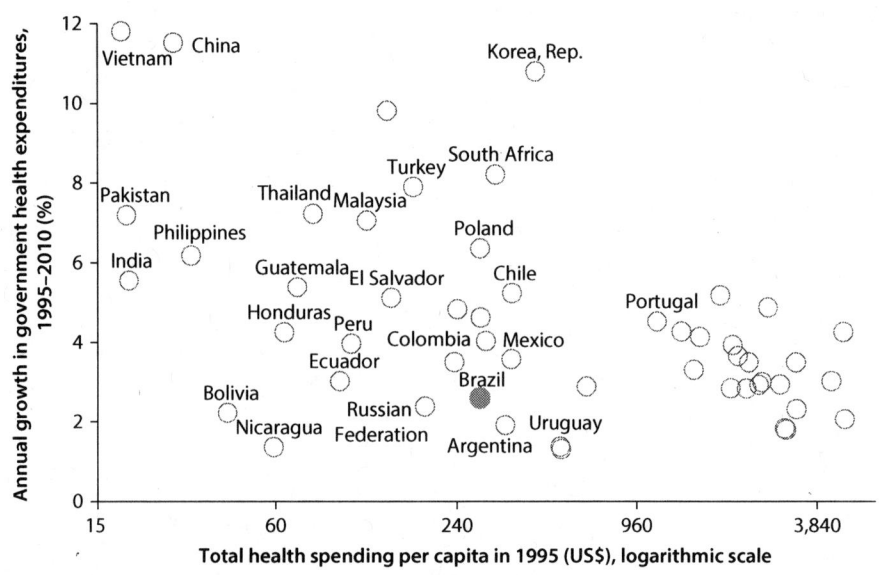

Source: Based on data from the World Health Organization (WHO) National Health Accounts (http:// www.who.int/nha).

Figure 2.18 Government Health Spending as a Percentage of GDP in Select Countries, 2010

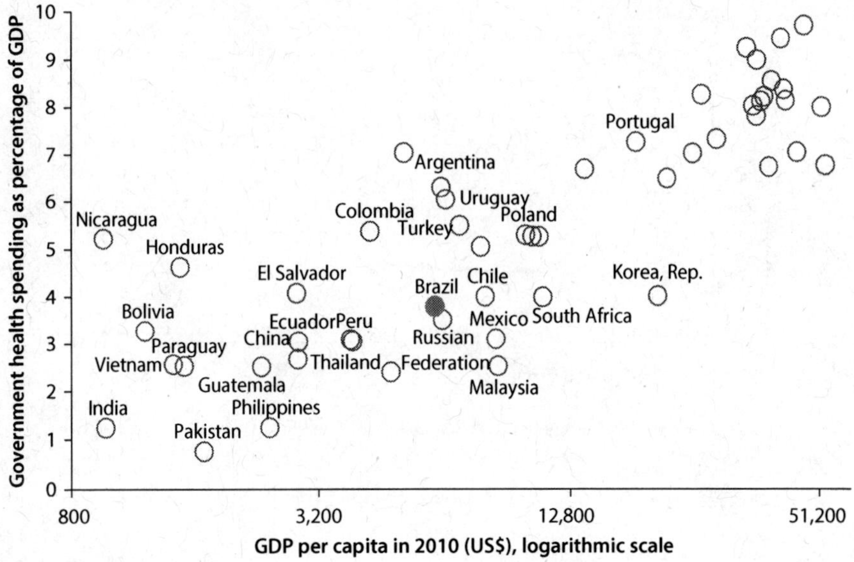

Source: Based on data from the World Health Organization (WHO) National Health Accounts (http://www.who.int/nha).
Note: GDP = gross domestic product.

Composition of Government Spending on Health

The expansion of the outpatient care network and the ESF was accompanied by a change in funding priorities, with primary care receiving an increasing share of federal funds (figure 2.19). Federal transfers for basic care increased proportionally between 1995 and 2002 (from 11 percent to around 20 percent of total transfers), but then stabilized at around 17 percent.[9] In constant (2010) per capita values, Ministry of Health spending on primary health care increased from R$27 in 1995 to R$50 in 2010.

The composition of spending also shifted at the state and municipal levels (figure 2.20). Municipal governments clearly spend the larger part of their health budget on primary care, while state governments spend a low and decreasing proportion on primary care (as much of this activity was transferred to municipalities); the proportion of federal budget spending on primary care is associated with transfers to municipalities, as the Ministry of Health has almost no responsibility for primary health care. However, the decline in the proportion of municipal spending on primary health care is due to the transfer of hospitals and outpatient referral facilities to local governments in association with the municipalization process.

It is difficult to estimate total SUS expenditure by these service categories over such a long period of time due to gaps or inconsistencies in the data. However, available data suggest that the proportion of government budget for health (health budget function) allocated to basic care (basic care sub function) increased steadily between the early 1970s and 2010, from 10 percent to around 20 percent. The increase is greater if public health and health surveillance are

Figure 2.19 Allocation of the Ministry of Health Budget in Brazil, by Type of Care, 1995–2010

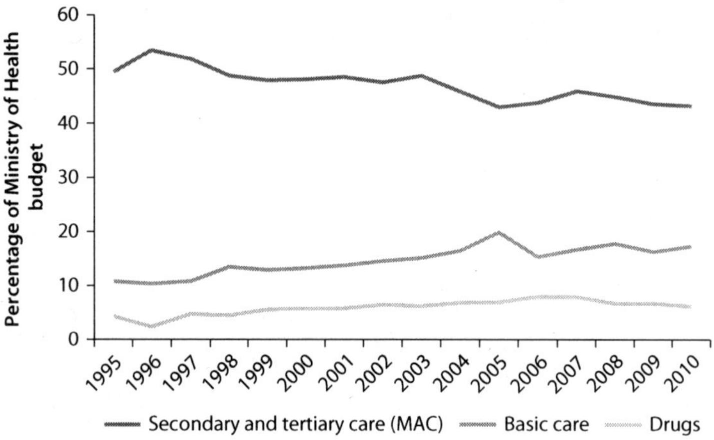

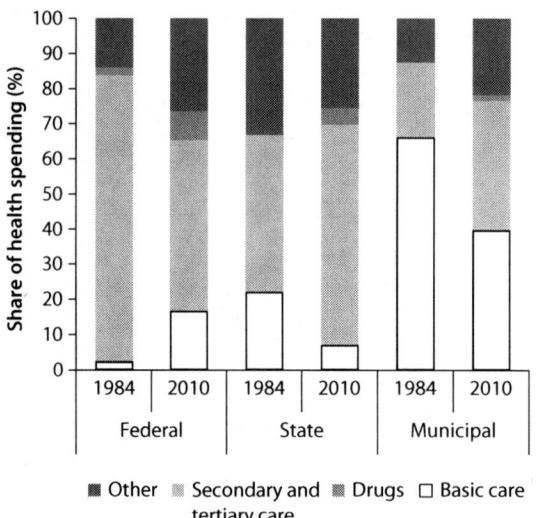

Source: Ministry of Health, DATASUS.
Note: MAC (*média e alta complexidade*) is a grouping of medium- and high-complexity services.

Figure 2.20 Allocation of Health Spending in Brazil, by Level of Government and Type of Care, 1984 and 2010

Source: Based on budget data from the Ministry of Health and the Ministry of Finance, STN 2010.
Note: The estimates may be biased because of inconsistencies and changes in expenditure classification and programs or activities included in "administrative and other."

added to primary care. But the importance of primary health care spending varies by level of government.

The reallocation of resources in favor of primary care has helped to reduce the hospital-centric nature of the existing system of the 1970s and 1980s. Nonetheless, hospital services continue to account for nearly half of government spending, and spending on the hospital sector has grown steadily despite a decrease in SUS admissions per capita. Some of this increase has been the result of investment in high-complexity services. Meanwhile, medium-complexity care, which provides the link between improved and expanded primary care and the successful high-complexity programs, has been identified as a major weakness in the SUS for several years (see, for example, Ministry of Health 2011). Indeed, general inpatient care and specialized outpatient care have received little attention, and this segment of the system is often unable to meet the increase in demand generated by the expansion of primary health care and the growing burden of chronic disease (Ministry of Health 2011).[10]

Financing Mix across Levels of Government

Reflecting the drastic decentralization of service delivery responsibilities, the financing mix by level of government changed notably over the last two decades (figure 2.21). During most of the 1980s, federal spending accounted for the larger part of public expenditure (74 percent on average) increasing to 85 percent in the years immediately preceding the formal creation of the SUS. Since then, the federal share has decreased steadily, reaching 45 percent in the late 2000s. In contrast, both municipal and state spending has increased steadily since 1988, reaching 28 and 27 percent, respectively, in 2009. This increase preceded the constitutional amendment in 2000, but has been more pronounced since.

This change in financing pattern was a clear result of the transfer of responsibilities to municipal governments. However, SUS analysts and supporters alike have criticized the stagnant level of federal spending as being inconsistent with the goals of the system. Moreover, many states and especially municipalities appear to have reached a level of financial contribution that is difficult to

Figure 2.21 Share of SUS Financing in Brazil, by Level of Government, 1980–2009

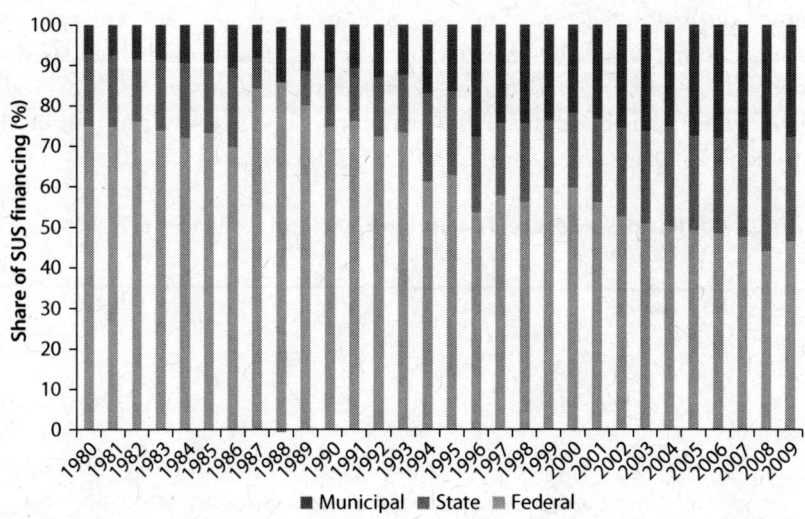

Sources: Based on Ministry of Health, SIOPS data; Medici 1991; Ministry of Finance, STN 2010.
Note: SUS = Sistema Único de Saúde.

Twenty Years of Health System Reform in Brazil • http://dx.doi.org/10.1596/978-0-8213-9843-2

increase further and maybe even to maintain (see, for example, Pereira *et al.*
2006; de Sousa and Hamann 2009; Macinko 2011).

Regional Disparities in Government Spending

While the SUS reforms did not increase government spending on health as much
as anticipated, they did manage to reduce disparities in government spending
significantly across states and municipalities. This was achieved not only by making targeted investments in expanding the health system in underserved parts of
the country, but also by changing the criteria for allocating federal and state funds
for health. Indeed, federal transfers were increasingly targeted toward the poorer
states of the Northeast and North: 5 of the 10 states with relatively large
increases in federal spending are in the Northeast and 3 are in the North. In the
richer states of the Southeast, South, and Center-West, only three states experienced an increase in federal spending (Espírito Santo, Mato Grosso do Sul, and
Santa Catarina). As a result, not only did the variation in spending per capita
decline (figure 2.22), but the relationship between a state's average income and
health spending also weakened over time (figure 2.23). Even so, significant
spending gaps remain, with spending per capita ranging from around R$500 in
Ceará, Maranhão, and Pará, to more than R$1,300 in Mato Grosso do Sul, Rio
Grande do Sul, and São Paulo.

Private Health Financing: Out-of-Pocket Payments and Private Insurance

Although the SUS reforms did not establish explicit goals for private spending,
the "supplemental" health system was expected to decline in importance as
the national health system expanded and matured. This did not happen.
Indeed, despite intentions to the contrary, private spending remained stable
over the last 15 years or so (from around 57 percent in 1995 to 54 percent of
total health spending in 2009; figure 2.24). The share of direct out-of-pocket
spending declined over time, but still accounts for around 30 percent of total
health spending, while the share of spending on private plans increased and
now stands at just over 20 percent. The number of individuals covered by
private health plans grew steadily over the last 20 years—by 2009, more than
50 million Brazilians were covered by some form of plan.

Figure 2.22 SUS Health Spending per Capita across States in Brazil, 1995 and 2009

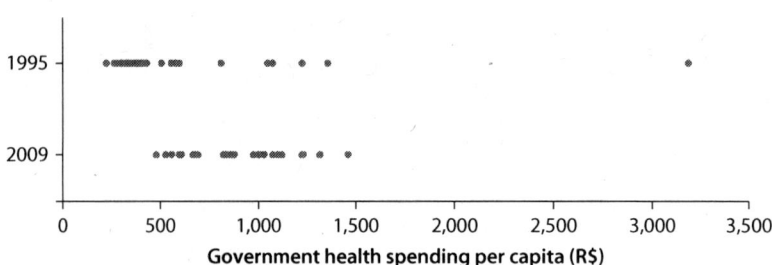

Source: Couttolenc 2011.
Note: SUS = Sistema Único de Saúde.

Figure 2.23 SUS Spending per Capita on Health and Average Monthly Income per Capita across States in Brazil, 1995 and 2009

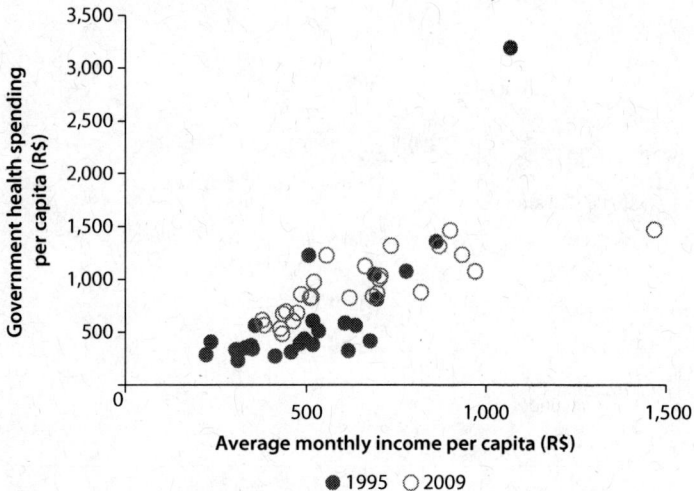

Sources: Couttolenc 2011; IPEAData (from IBGE) for state income levels.
Note: SUS = Sistema Único de Saúde.

Figure 2.24 Share of Private Health Spending in Total Health Spending in Brazil, 1995–2009

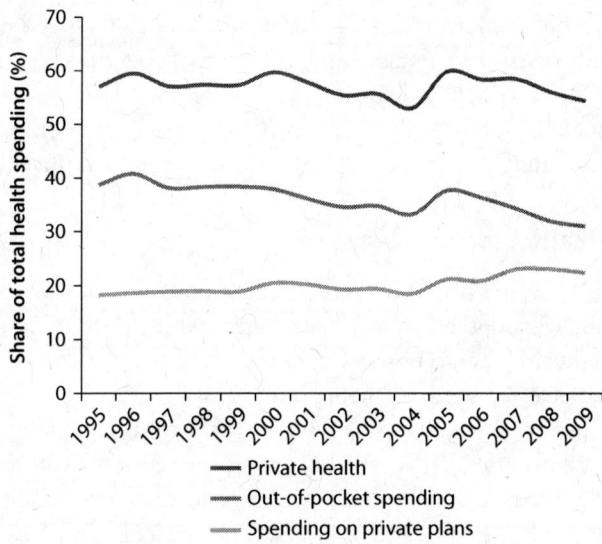

Source: Based on data from the WHO National Health Accounts (http:// www.who.int/nha).

As a result of the continued growth in private spending, the share of total health spending financed by government in Brazil is significantly lower than what is observed in OECD countries and in many middle-income peers (figure 2.25). For instance, in Colombia, Thailand, and Turkey, all of which established universal health coverage over the last couple of decades, government spending accounts

Figure 2.25 Government Financing of Health Expenditures in Select Countries, by GDP per Capita, 2010

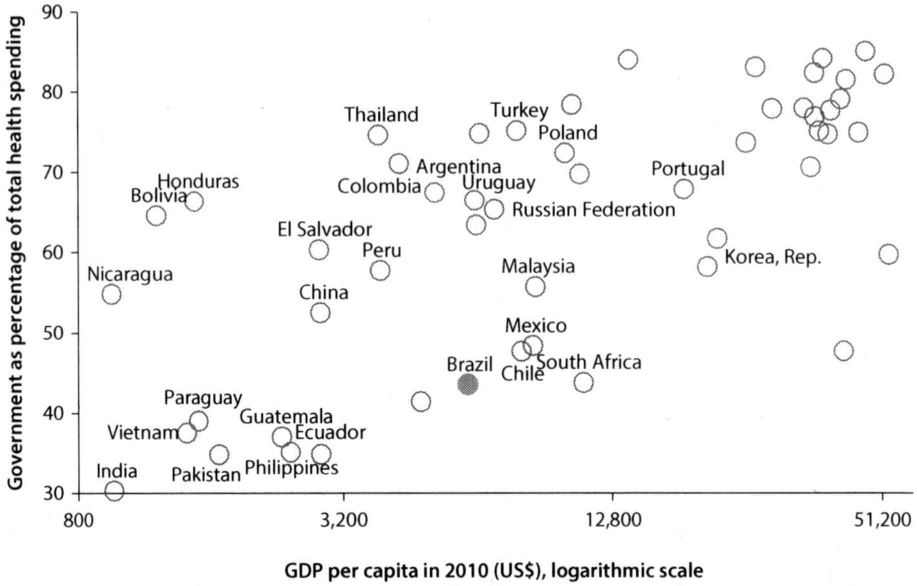

Source: Based on data from the WHO National Health Accounts (http:// www.who.int/nha).
Note: GDP = gross domestic product.

for somewhere between 70 and 75 percent of total health spending, compared with around 45 percent in Brazil. Although part of this private spending is for private health plans, which, at least in principle, provide some protection against high out-of-pocket spending, the high share of private spending has important implications for equity and fairness of both access to care and financing burden.[11]

Enhancing Health System Governance

Although the SUS reforms did not articulate explicit goals or principles for governance and accountability, these concepts were implicit in many of the changes to the health system that the reforms envisaged. For the purposes of this report, governance is seen as being concerned with the management of relationships between various stakeholders in health, including individuals, households, communities, firms, levels of governments, nongovernmental organizations, private firms, and other entities that have the responsibility to finance, monitor, deliver, and use health services. The systems and institutions that manage these relationships can have a profound impact on the performance of the health system.

Although this report does not undertake a comprehensive assessment of health system governance in Brazil, it highlights several questions for which the SUS reforms have significant implications for governance. First, to what extent has the universal right to health care established by the 1998 Constitution been operationalized (and can be operationalized), and what are the main legal consequences associated with it? Second, to what extent have adequate institutions and systems for financing and intergovernmental coordination been developed to meet the needs of the drastic decentralization of service responsibilities? Third, have the principles of participation and voice been translated effectively into reality? Finally, has there been sufficient innovation in the way that the government provides and pays for services to ensure that improvements in efficiency, effectiveness, and integration are realized?[12]

Establishment and Consequences of the Right to Health

Establishing the universal right to health was a key element of the SUS and the movement leading to it. It emerged from the democratic movements that led to the country's democratization in the early to mid-1980s, and in that sense it was a political and social achievement rather than a technical decision. The right to health progressed on two fronts during the 1970s and 1980s: politically, by being a key aspiration of the democratization movement that began in the late 1970s, leading to the first presidential election in 1985 and to the Constitution of 1988, and technically, by gradually bringing different social groups (rural workers and informal workers) under Social Security to provide a stronger basis for the "Brazilian economic miracle" of the 1970s. In the mid-1980s, several National Health Conferences (especially that of 1986) strengthened the movement, and the requirement to show that one contributed to the Social Security system in order to receive care within the INAMPS system was dropped. Finally, all of this culminated in establishing the constitutional right to health. However, as a mostly political process, the decision to grant universal and free coverage to health care was not accompanied by a discussion of the resources needed to support it.

The right to health was confirmed in the basic legislation of the SUS, published in 1990 (the Health Organic Law/Law 8.080 and Law 8.142), which merely repeated the statements in the Constitution that "the state should provide the necessary conditions for its full exercise," through economic and social policies to reduce health risks and efforts to ensure the "conditions" for universal and equitable access. The extensive regulations published over the following years provided no strategy or guidance on how to operationalize this right. In 2006, the Ministry of Health published a Chart of Health Rights, which proposed explicit and operational principles and guidelines for the rights to health care.

Indirectly, although not formally, the right to health was operationalized through two general principles: first, by legally ensuring that anyone can be treated for free under the SUS and, second, by expanding the public network of health facilities and services to make those services accessible. In fact, neither of these two principles is a necessary condition to ensure the right to health care, since health services do not need to be free or provided within a public system to be accessible. In several countries where the right to health care is considered to be guaranteed and universal, health services are not free (they are subsidized) and are not necessarily provided by a public system (coverage may be mandated rather than provided, as in the Netherlands). Moreover, by not offering an explicit list of covered services (and therefore implicitly covering all services needed by a sick person), the SUS is more generous, at least on paper, than the systems in most developed and rich countries, which have regulated and defined a list of covered services and the conditions or circumstances under which they are covered. For instance, countries such as Canada and the United Kingdom limit or prioritize the coverage of certain expensive procedures to cases in which the patient is most likely to benefit from them (along a cost-effectiveness principle).

A significant contradiction between the universal right to health and the access to health services it implies lies in the fact that, in spite of the open-ended service package, the SUS pays or reimburses providers for a limited list of services. Moreover, the open-ended benefits package is unlikely to be enforceable in a sustained manner, a contradiction that has generated two important legal conflicts.

First, many patients seek to obtain expensive drugs or treatments that are not yet included on the SUS list by seeking a legal injunction. Such mandates represent an increasing and significant burden on SUS finances, while not necessarily providing clear benefits to patients. They also tend to create inequalities, as rich patients are more likely to be aware of new procedures and treatments that are available internationally and to go to court to obtain them.

Second, private insurers challenge in court the requirement to reimburse the SUS for the cost of services provided to SUS enrollees, based on the principle of universal coverage. Moreover, the absence of a clear list of covered services and goods allows providers to expand the supply and use of expensive new technologies. This has been shown to be an important source of inefficiencies and unnecessary costs, as Brazil has been quick to adopt new technologies and allocates them in an inefficient way.

The SUS has recently undertaken significant efforts to face these challenges, in particular with respect to incorporating new technologies and establishing a dialogue with the courts. In the first case, the Ministry of Health has established an internal unit to develop guidelines for assessing new technologies and including them in SUS lists. In the latter case, health authorities are developing a dialogue with the courts to ensure that judges consider the technical and cost implications of new technologies when ruling on a claimant's request.

Institutions for Coordination and Financing across Levels of Government

As a result of the SUS reforms, the provision of most primary health services and nearly half of hospital care has been transferred to municipal governments. Decentralization has been achieved to a large extent, even though the degree of decentralization of facilities and resources varies substantially across states. The drastic shift in responsibility for financing and delivery to lower levels of government required the development of new mechanisms for coordination and negotiation across autonomous levels of government, in particular because these had been a key weakness of the pre-SUS system.

Much effort was spent in the early years of the SUS to design and implement basic legislation and internal management mechanisms, leading to the establishment of bilateral and trilateral committees in 1993.[13] With these institutional innovations, coordination improved, and many of the pre-SUS problems of duplication and fragmentation were resolved. However, these mechanisms have proved bureaucratic and cumbersome, with unclear assignment of decision-making power leading to slow and inefficient planning and budgeting processes and high transaction costs.

On the financing side, payment mechanisms evolved over time, both for intergovernmental transfers and for payments to providers. Transfers were initially made directly to providers based on service volume (outpatient and inpatient care); starting in the early 1990s, they became conditional on a set of formal administrative and financial requirements, globally known as SUS accreditation of states and municipalities. In order to provide incentives for states and municipalities to implement or expand national policies and programs, specific transfers were linked to specific programs.

The second half of the decade saw a major change in transfer mechanisms, when comprehensive block grants were devised to finance the expansion of primary care. Two parallel mechanisms were implemented: (a) the Basic Care Grant (*Piso da Atenção Básica*), based on a monthly amount per capita to finance most decentralized public health programs and activities, and (b) the payment mechanism to finance strategic primary health care programs, especially the ESF and the PACS.[14] However, in order to provide incentives to implement or expand specific programs, the Ministry of Health multiplied the number of payment mechanisms to an unmanageable number: in 2002, more than 100 transfer mechanisms were in place. More recently, they were grouped into five broad block grants: basic care, medium- and high-complexity care, health surveillance, pharmaceutical care, and SUS management. However, many of the original payment mechanisms are still maintained as formulas making up the five blocks.

Over most of the 1990s and early 2000s, a conflict raged between unconditional federal transfers (fund-to-fund) and transfers linked to service volume or program targets. On the one hand, because subnational governments are fully autonomous under Brazil's federal system, they see conditional transfers as an undue interference from the Ministry of Health in regional and local allocation of resources and health system management. On the other hand, the federal government sees conditional transfers as a means of stimulating and guiding implementation of the SUS and national health policies. In the early 1990s, as the SUS was implemented and regulated, emphasis was placed on transfers conditional on states and municipalities meeting administrative and financial criteria to be "accredited" for SUS implementation. In the mid-1990s, transfers for primary care started, including a variable incentive linked to negotiated program and service targets and coverage by the PACS and the ESF. Later, the proportion of unconditional fund-to-fund transfers gradually increased.

More generally, the decentralization process has raised questions about the capacity of states and municipalities to perform designated functions (box 2.3)

Box 2.3 Assessing Local Capacity to Manage Decentralized Responsibilities

A pilot survey of state-level capacity to manage the Sistema Único de Saúde (SUS) was undertaken in 2005–06 under the coordination of the National Council of State Secretaries of Health (Conselho Nacional de Secretários de Saúde, CONASS), using the Pan American Health Organization's framework for assessing essential public health functions (CONASS and OPAS 2007). The report, covering five states (Ceará, Goias, Mato Grosso, Rondônia, and Sergipe), assessed each state's infrastructure, institutional capacity, processes, and outcomes in performing the essential functions. Using a participatory approach, it measured overall performance on a scale of 0–1.

The mean scale for the five states was only 0.55, varying between 0.43 and 0.63 (table B2.3.1). But the score for specific functions varied widely. The stronger essential functions among the five states were coordination (F11) and policy, planning, and management (F5), while the weakest were health promotion and quality (F9), promotion of universal access (F7), and human resources (F8). Most of the functions associated with outcomes (F7, F9) had poor ratings, while those associated with SUS administrative processes had better ones. This is not surprising given the early emphasis on administrative processes and formal requirements during SUS implementation. However, the instrument was applied to smaller states with relatively weaker institutional capacity, although at least two of them (Ceará and Sergipe) have recent initiatives related to the organization and delivery of health care; overall, the survey findings are not necessarily representative of the situation and capacity in the majority of states.

Some process indicators also describe the extent to which state governments achieve SUS regulatory requirements: (a) SUS health agreements signed by a state and its municipalities;

Table B2.3.1 Performance Scores for Essential Public Health Functions of Five State Secretariats in Brazil, 2006

Function	Mean	Range
F1. Monitoring, analysis, and evaluation of health situation in the state	0.54	0.46–0.59
F2. Surveillance, investigation, and control of risks and harms to health	0.64	0.50–0.76
F3. Health promotion	0.52	0.43–0.67
F4. Social participation in health	0.54	0.37–0.70
F5. Policy development and institutional capacity for planning and public management of health	0.71	0.57–0.86
F6. Capacity for regulation, oversight, control, and audit in health	0.56	0.22–0.70
F7. Promotion and guarantee of universal and equitable access to health services	0.47	0.33–0.58
F8. Human resources management, development, and formation	0.38	0.08–0.55
F9. Promotion and guarantee of quality in health services	0.31	0.09–0.51
F10. Research and technology incorporation in health	0.55	0.39–0.80
F11. Coordination of the regionalization and decentralization process in health	0.79	0.72–0.91
Final score	0.55	0.43–0.63

Source: CONASS and OPAS 2007.
Note: The states covered are Ceará, Goias, Mato Grosso, Rondônia, and Sergipe.

box continues next page

Box 2.3 Assessing Local Capacity to Manage Decentralized Responsibilities *(continued)*

(b) up-to-date planning documents (state health plan and integrated planning and programming document); (c) establishment and coverage of regional health councils, a recent strategy to strengthen regionalization; (d) approval of annual management reports by state and municipal health councils; and (e) implementation of a contracting instrument with private providers and the proportion of providers covered.

These indicators varied widely across states. The best achievers were Bahia, Mato Grosso do Sul, Paraná, São Paulo, and Tocantins, while the worst were Maranhão, Piauí, Roraima, and—a surprising finding—Rio Grande do Sul. While some of these responsibilities are conducted at the municipal level, a strong and active state secretariat of health can help municipalities under its jurisdiction to achieve better functions, especially in implementing SUS regulations.

---

and about whether some of the 5,600 municipalities that now have primary responsibility for delivering health services are too small to achieve economies of scale and scope in managing the health system. Reflecting this concern, there are ongoing efforts to define a new level of organization of the system: regional health networks that sit between the state and municipal levels. This idea dates back to the 1980s, but became an official policy in early 2000, when the SUS Health Care Operational Guideline (Regulations 01/2001 and 01/2002) identified implementation of a "hierarchical and regionalized health system" as a key objective.

Several disease-specific networks were defined in the early 2000s (cardiology, transplants, burns, emergency care), and some of them were successfully implemented, such as the Mobile Emergency Service (Sistema de Assistência Médica de Urgência, SAMU). More recently, the Ministry of Health is seeking to develop and implement networks based on treatment guidelines for specific types of care, including hypertension, diabetes, cancer, and perinatal mortality, and ongoing initiatives are seeking to establish regional networks organized around new intermunicipal organizations.[15] However, very few functional networks have been put in place so far, and integrated care networks remain one of the major challenges for improving SUS effectiveness and overall performance.

Social Participation and Voice

Democratization in the health system has been a major objective of the health reforms, and mechanisms for ensuring the democratization of decision making, planning, and evaluation within the SUS have been a major feature of the new system. In the early 1980s, the public health system not only was centralized, with little participation and decision-making power at the state and municipal levels, but also reflected the authoritarian rule of the military regime that ended in 1985. The health councils that were established at each level—federal, state, and municipal—provide formal mechanisms for society participation and voice and include representatives from health authorities, health professionals, providers, and users. However, their effectiveness varies greatly; in many cases, they end up being rubber-stamping entities or being captured by political interests (see, for instance, Paim *et al.* 2011).

Purchaser-Provider Relationships

On the provider side, the last 20 years has seen a slow but steady shift away from contracting services from private hospitals and toward providing services through public hospitals. This shift has been accompanied by some limited changes in how the SUS finances or purchases services. In the early 1980s, most payments to private hospitals were done on the basis of fee-for-service, which produced substantial inefficiencies and distortions. Public providers, in contrast, were financed on the basis of traditional line-item budgets. The system was improved in the early 1980s, with computerization and the adoption of automatic checks and controls to identify errors and fraud (La Forgia and Couttolenc 2008). For inpatient care, fee-for-service was replaced by a prospective payment mechanism based on medical procedures known as the authorization for hospital admission (*autorização de internação hospitalar*, AIH). As shown in La Forgia and Couttolenc (2008), this represented a major improvement over the previous fee-for-service system, but became gradually and increasingly distorted by the absence of systematic revisions and reliable information on costs.

In parallel to the early rounds of payment reform, several initiatives have been undertaken to develop new organizational models for delivering services. Early efforts focused on transforming hospitals into public foundations and public enterprises. Some of these initiatives were successfully implemented, but have proved difficult to replicate. More recently, São Paulo State started contracting private not-for-profit organizations—known as social organizations (*organizações sociais*)—to deliver health services, and other states and municipalities have followed suit. Under this model, facility managers have significant autonomy, but also explicit contractual obligations (box 2.4). However, concern over facility governance, remuneration, and performance has been gaining strength more broadly. This concern has translated into new contracting arrangements between the SUS and university and nonprofit hospitals and into new legislation regarding public foundations.

Although limited in scale, new provider models have resulted in innovative payment and contracting arrangements. For instance, São Paulo State uses performance-based contracts to purchase hospital services from social organizations, and Rio de Janeiro Municipality uses a similar model to contract both hospital services and primary care services (family clinics). While the São Paulo model has been deemed successful, there is less evidence on performance in other parts of the country. However, capacity in contract design and monitoring is often a significant constraint.

Overall, innovations in organizational models, provider payment, and contracting are limited, but gaining momentum. Many of these innovations hold promise, but it will be important to evaluate the reforms carefully, looking both at the extent to which they are achieving intended results and at the conditions required for effective implementation. Only with this information can informed

---

Box 2.4 The Social Organization Model in São Paulo State

Based on the state reform framework proposed in 1995 and legally established by Federal Law 9637 of 1998, a social organization is a fully autonomous entity managed by a certified nonprofit organization to provide social services on behalf of the state. The São Paulo State legislature immediately passed a law adapting the federal law, and the state government went on to implement the new model. It was initially applied to 11 newly built hospitals, where the new (private) managers hired staff based on the Private Employment Law.

Six features characterized the model as implemented in São Paulo: (a) state ownership of buildings and equipment; (b) private management by a certified social organization with recognized experience in hospital management; (c) public funding, but full financial and managerial autonomy; (d) management contract signed by the government and the social organization, with clear objectives, goals, and measurable targets; (e) staff hired under private law; and (f) strong oversight and contract management from the state secretariat of health.

La Forgia and Couttolenc (2008) demonstrated that the São Paulo social organizations performed significantly better than similar hospitals under typical public management. Their score for technical efficiency, which was computed using data envelopment analysis, was 50 percent higher, reaching a level of efficiency comparable to that of private facilities under corporate (for-profit) governance. They also had higher indicators of productivity and quality than a control group of public hospitals. After controlling for several factors, Matzuda *et al.* (2008) identified key factors contributing to the difference in performance, including a strong accountability mechanism between provider (social organizations) and purchaser (state secretariat of health). This mechanism included performance-based contracting and the ability of managers to hire and fire personnel and thus define the appropriate mix of staff skills, which in turn improves staff motivation.

In 2011, São Paulo Municipality deployed a broad strategy for improving autonomy and governance at the facility level. It includes establishing and contracting with social organizations to manage 5 hospitals, 15 emergency centers, and 5 diagnostic services in a model similar to that of São Paulo State, signing management contracts with 327 primary health care facilities, contracting with social organizations to manage regional networks, and establishing public-private partnerships for constructing, expanding, and managing four new hospitals.

Source: La Forgia and Couttolenc 2008.

---

decisions be made about what models may be appropriate for the very diverse conditions in Brazil's states and municipalities.

Notes

1. Law 8.080 states that the private sector is free to participate in the delivery of health services, provided that it complies with ethical norms and government regulations. Furthermore, the law includes provisions for the SUS to rely on private services in cases where adequate converge cannot be ensured, with preference given

to philanthropic or other nonprofit organizations. The law prohibits the SUS from subsidizing or providing financial support to private for-profit providers.

2. The PACS covered about 16 million people in 1994, before the ESF was launched, mostly in the states of Bahia, Ceará, and Maranhão. These areas reached high levels of coverage (above 70 percent) in the early 2000s.

3. The Family Health Strategy was initially known as the Family Health Program. For simplicity, this report calls it the Family Health Strategy or ESF throughout.

4. ESF "enrollment" is not based on individual choice; it is determined by whether a person's residence is within the ESF team's catchment area. In heavily populated areas, there may be more than one ESF team per health facility, but each team is assigned a specific territory and has a list of which families it serves. Hence, in this report, we refer to "ESF enrollees" as those people whose household is within the catchment area of an ESF basic care unit and who therefore are on the list of families for which that ESF unit is responsible. As with other services delivered by the SUS, there are no user fees for services and most medications are delivered free of charge.

5. During 2002–06, expansion of the ESF in larger municipalities occurred at the same pace as in smaller municipalities. The World Bank Family Health Strategy Project, which aimed to expand coverage and strengthen the ESF in 187 large municipalities (with more than 100,000 people), may have contributed to this trend (Ministry of Health 2008; Facchini *et al.* 2006).

6. According to a Ministry of Health study, nearly two-thirds of ESF team professionals in 2002 had been hired under temporary or short-term contracts (Ministry of Health, CGPRH and Universidade Federal de Minas Gerais, NESCON 2002).

7. The national systems (Ministry of Health, Ministry of Education, and INAMPS) were largely merged into one system, which in turn was integrated with state and municipal systems (university hospitals continue to be managed by the Ministry of Education, but are formally part of the SUS).

8. The series on government health spending are not fully consistent over time. In particular, there have been some changes in the treatment of government spending for civil servants, the military, and teaching hospitals under the Ministry of Education. Moreover, the expenditure data do not reflect subsidies to the private sector. However, these gaps and inconsistencies in the data do not significantly change the overall trend.

9. In 2002, there was a break in the series when transfer and payment mechanisms were regrouped into five transfer blocks.

10. Some successful experiences of the ESF in larger municipalities have emphasized restructuring the organization of and access to specialized care based on the Family Health Strategy (Giovanella *et al.* 2009; Macinko 2011).

11. This issue is discussed in more detail in chapter 3.

12. These are not the only aspects of governance and accountability that are relevant to the health sector. The last 20 years also saw significant measures to strengthen consumer protection (for example, the establishment of PROCON, a consumer protection agency), improve monitoring and reporting, and strengthen an increasingly proactive Federal Audit Tribunal (Tribunal de Contas de União), to mention a few. The report does not get into these broader institutional reforms.

13. Bilateral committees operate in each state and include representatives of state and municipal health authorities (state and municipal health secretariats); the trilateral committee also includes representatives from the Ministry of Health.

14. Financing was linked to the number of ESF teams in place and coverage of the PACS. This incentive was instrumental in the rapid deployment of the two programs.

15. The municipalities of Aracaju, Belo Horizonte, and Curitiba, for instance, have often been cited as successful and interesting models, but little systematic analytical work has been done on the issue (one exception is Matzuda et al. 2008, which analyzes the Curitiba experience). The implementation of local or regional health care networks focusing on guidelines for care is the subject of the ongoing Qualisus-Rede Project funded by the World Bank (see Ministry of Health 2006; World Bank 2007).

References

CONASS (Conselho Nacional de Secretários de Saúde) and OPAS (Organização Pan-Americana de Saúde). 2007. A gestão da saúde nos estados: Avaliação e fortalecimento das funções essenciais. Brasilia.

Couttolenc, B. 2011. "Taking Stock of Performance Reforms at the Sub-National Level in Brazil: Recent Performance Gains Achieved in the Health Sector, Hypotheses on Possible Drivers of Good and Bad Performance." Consultant report, World Bank, Washington, DC.

de Sousa, M., and E. Hamann. 2009. "Programa Saúde da Família no Brasil: Uma agenda incompleta?" Cien Saúde Coletiva 14 (Suppl 1): 1325–35.

Facchini, L., R. Piccini, E. Tomasi, E. Thumé, D. Silveira, F. Siqueira, and M. Rodrigues. 2006. "Desempenho do PSF no sul e no nordeste do Brasil: Avaliação institucional e epidemiológica da atenção básica à saúde." Universidade de Pelotas, Ciência & Saúde Coletiva 11 (3): 669–81.

Giovanella, L., M. Mendonça, P. de Almeida, S. Escorel, C. Senna Mde, M. Fausto, M. Delgado, C. de Andrade, M. da Cunha, M. Martins, and C. Teixeira. 2009. "Family Health: Limits and Possibilities for an Integral Primary Care Approach to Health Care in Brazil." Cien Saúde Coletiva 14 (3): 783–94.

IBGE (Instituto Brasileiro de Geografia e Estatística). 2008. Pesquisa nacional por amostragem de domicilios. Rio de Janeiro: IBGE.

———. 2010. Estatísticas da saúde: Assistência médico-sanitária (AMS) 2009. Rio de Janeiro: IBGE.

Iglesias, R., P. Jha, M. Pinto, V. L. C. Silva, and J. Godinho. 2007. "Controle do tabagismo no Brasil." HNP Discussion Paper, World Bank, Washington, DC.

La Forgia, G. M., and B. F. Couttolenc. 2008. Hospital Performance in Brazil: In Search of Excellence. Washington, DC: World Bank.

Macinko, J. 2011. "A Preliminary Assessment of the Family Health Strategy (FHS) in Brazil." Consultant report, World Bank, Washington, DC.

Matzuda, Y., J. Rinne, G. Shepherd, and G. Wenceslau. 2008. "Brazil: Enhancing Performance in Brazil's Health Sector: Lessons from Innovations in the State of São Paulo and the City of Curitiba." Brief Note 116, World Bank, Washington, DC, February.

Medici, A. C. 1991. Perspectivas do financiamento à saúde no governo Collor de Mello. Série Economia e Financiamento 2. Brasilia: OPAS.

Ministry of Finance, STN (National Treasury Secretariat). 2010. "Orçamentos fiscal e da seguridade social." Série Histórica da Consolidação das Contas Públicas, Brasilia.

Ministry of Health. 2006. "QUALISUS: Projeto de investimentos para a qualificação do Sistema Único de Saúde." Documento do Projeto Revisado, Brasilia.

———. 2008. *Saúde da família no Brasil: Uma análise de indicadores selecionados, 1998–2005/06.* Brasilia.

———. 2011. "Programa de avaliação para a qualificação do Sistema Único de Saúde." Ministério da Saúde, Secretaria Executiva, Brasilia.

Ministry of Health, CGPRH (Coordenação Geral de Políticas de Recursos Humanos) and Universidade Federal de Minas Gerais, NESCON (Núcleo de Educação em Saúde Coletiva). 2002. "Agentes institucionais e modalidades de contratação de pessoal no Programa de Saúde da Família no Brasil." Relatorio de Pesquisa, Universidade Federal de Minas Gerais, Belo Horizonte.

Ministry of Health, DAB (Departamento do Atenção Básica). 2011. "Performance Data on the Family Health Program." Ministério da Saúde, Brasilia. http://dab.saude.gov.br/abnumeros.php.

Paim, J., C. Travassos, C. Almeida, and J. Macinko. 2011. "O sistema de saúde brasileiro: História, avanços e desafios." Série Saúde no Brasil 1, *thelancet.com* (May 9): 11–31.

Pereira, A., A. de Sá Campelo, F. Cunha, J. Noronha, H. Cordeiro, S. Dain, and T. Pereira. 2006. "The Economic-Financial Sustainability of the PROESF in the States of Amapá, Maranhão, Pará, and Tocantins." *Cien Saúde Coletiva* 11 (3): 607–20.

Rocha, R., and R. Soares. 2009. "Evaluating the Impact of Community-Based Health Interventions: Evidence from Brazil's Family Health Program." Discussion Paper 4119, IZA, Bonn, Germany.

Schmidt, M., B. Duncan, G. Azevedo e Silva, A. Menezes, C. Monteiro, S. Barreto, D. Chor, and P. Menezes. 2011. "Chronic Non-Communicable Diseases in Brazil: Burden and Current Challenges." *thelancet.com* 377 (May 9): 1949–61.

World Bank. 2007. "Health Network Formation and Quality Improvement Project (Qualisus-Rede)." Project Appraisal Document, World Bank, Washington, DC.

Have the SUS Reforms Led to Better Outcomes?

While the Unified Health System (Sistema Único de Saúde, SUS) reforms focused on transforming how the health system is financed and organized, the ultimate goal was to universalize access to health services. This chapter assesses the extent to which this goal has been achieved. It also looks at progress in relation to other intermediate goals, in particular, with regard to quality and efficiency. It then turns to achievements in meeting the ultimate goals of the health system: improving health outcomes, reducing the financial burden of health expenditures, and enhancing trust in and satisfaction with the system. In doing so, it looks at how the SUS interfaces with private financing, the trends and patterns in the volume of services provided by the SUS and the utilization of services by households, and out-of-pocket payments on health. Beyond indicators related to coverage, the chapter also looks at trends in health outcomes and the extent to which improvements in health can be attributed to the SUS.

Use of Health Services and Progress toward Universality

Universality was a key founding principle of the SUS. Universal access or coverage is typically understood to mean that all people have access to a full spectrum of services without suffering undue financial hardship. Formally, the SUS reforms achieved this goal by decree: the Constitution and supporting legislation define health as a right, and all Brazilian citizens are entitled to have their health needs met by the SUS. To what extent has this formal entitlement translated into increased access and enhanced financial protection in practice?

Given the inherent imprecision in the definition of "universal coverage," this question is difficult to answer. What should be included in a "full spectrum of services"? At what point does the financial contribution required to pay for services become a "hardship"? There is no precise answer to these questions—coverage is inevitably a matter of degree. Nonetheless, we can derive at least a partial picture of how coverage has evolved by piecing together data from various sources on the use of health services and spending on health.

SUS "Coverage" and Fragmentation of the Health System

In assessing coverage of the SUS, the first question to answer is who is the system intended for? In 1981, 49 percent of the population reported that Social Security or the National Institute for Social Medical Assistance (Instituto Nacional de Assistência Médica da Previdência Social, INAMPS) was their "regular source of care," while another 19 percent relied on the public system or free philanthropic services (5 and 14 percent, respectively).[1] In other words, around 68 percent of the population relied on the elements of the system that were merged into the SUS in 1988. The remainder either used private health insurance (10 percent) or paid out-of-pocket for services delivered mostly by private providers (20 percent).

Implicit in the universality principle was the notion that most of the population relying on private health insurance and paying for their own health care would be brought into the integrated public system. If measured based on self-reported "regular sources of care," this goal has not been achieved. Indeed, by 2008, only 58 percent of individuals reported that they regularly use the SUS— lower than in 1981—while 26 and 19 percent reported that they rely primarily on private health insurance and pay for their care out-of-pocket, respectively.[2]

While this decline in the share of population indicating that the public systems are their regular source of care is significant, the picture is less clear when we look carefully at the patterns of use. In the same way that any regular users of the SUS sometimes pay for some services in the private sector, many who typically pay through private health insurance or pay out-of-pocket occasionally turn to the SUS. Indeed, some researchers argue that nearly all Brazilians use SUS services at some point. A 2003 survey lends credence to this view: it found that 28.6 percent of Brazilians were exclusive users of the SUS, 61.5 percent used both the SUS and other systems, and only 8.7 percent never used SUS services (CONASS 2003). More recent evidence suggests that reliance on the SUS increased over the last decade, with 60 percent indicating that they only use the public system (CNI 2012; figure 3.1), but these differences may be due at least in part to how the questions were asked.

Other evidence suggests that individuals "pick and choose" service providers, depending on the type of service and their circumstances. For instance, individuals use the SUS as the main source of both primary care (community health worker activities, immunizations, and some outpatient procedures) and more expensive services (hospitalization and high-cost therapies such as chemotherapy, radiation, and dialysis), but use private financing for general consultations, dental care, and diagnostic procedures (figure 3.2).

Even if most Brazilians use the SUS at some point, the apparent decline in the share of those who use the system as their regular source of care is significant. The fact that private health insurance and out-of-pocket expenditures continue to account for a large share of total health spending indicates that coverage gaps are present in the SUS or that concerns about quality and convenience lead those who can afford to pay privately for services to do so.

Figure 3.1 Use of Private and Public Providers of Health Care in Brazil, 2012

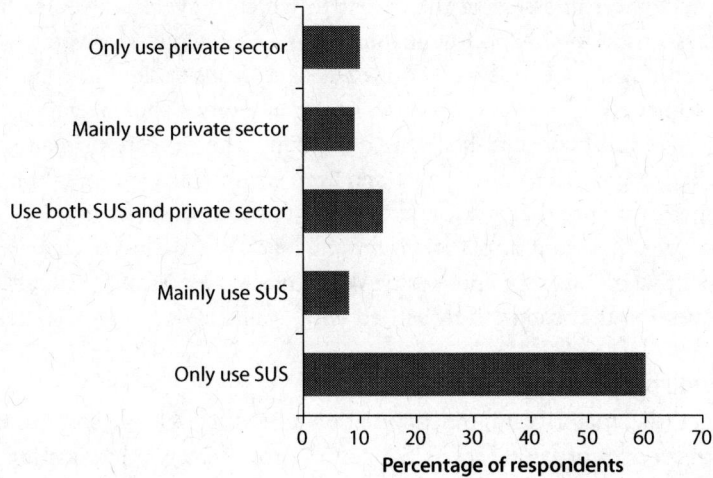

Source: CNI 2012.
Note: SUS = Sistema Único de Saúde.

Figure 3.2 Main Source of Care in Brazil, by Type of Service, 2008

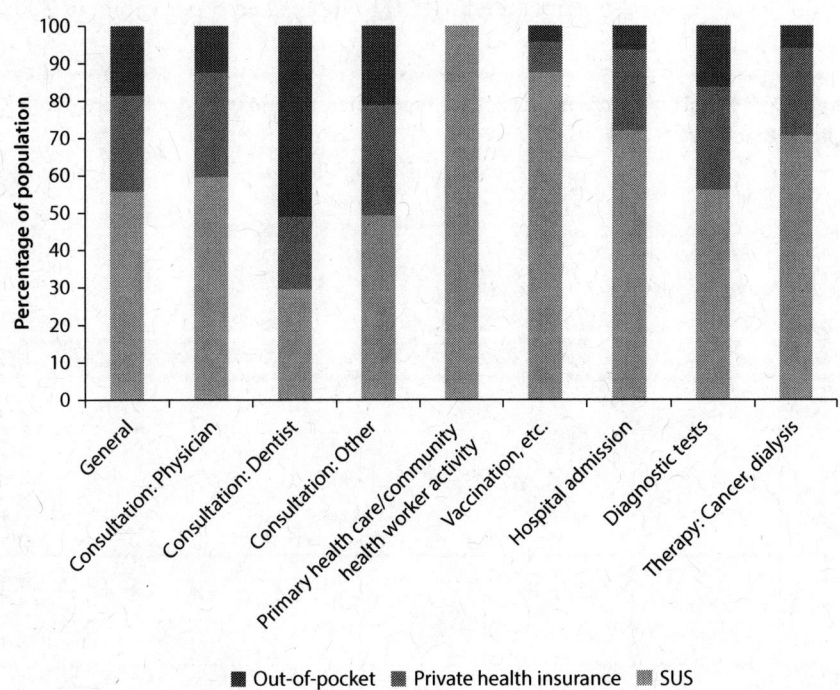

Source: IBGE, PNAD for 2008.
Note: SUS = Sistema Único de Saúde.

What is the nature of these coverage gaps or quality issues? This is a critical question to answer in assessing the extent to which universal coverage has been achieved. If, on the one hand, the inability to pay for services privately (through private health insurance or directly out-of-pocket) leads to significant inequalities in access to necessary care and eventual health outcomes, the coverage gaps are a matter of significant concern. If, on the other hand, the gaps are primarily in areas with limited implications for health and well-being (for example, brand name versus generic drugs or diagnostic and treatment procedures with limited efficacy), they may have important implications for efficiency, but are less of a concern from the perspective of coverage and equity. We return to this issue below, although it is not a question that can be fully settled with available data and evidence.

The Volume of Services Provided by SUS

Given that the majority of the population uses the SUS at some point, the volume of services provided by SUS facilities provides a good indication of realized access. The expansion of the network of facilities over the last two decades, documented in the previous chapter, has been accompanied by a large increase in the supply of services by the public system—INAMPS and then the SUS. The number of medical consultations per capita increased 70 percent between 1990 and 2009 (figure 3.3), and the volume of basic care procedures increased even more—from around 2.5 per capita in 1990 to more than 8 per capita in 2009.[3]

Figure 3.3 Medical Consultations, Basic Care Procedures, and Hospital Admissions per Capita in Brazil, 1980–2009

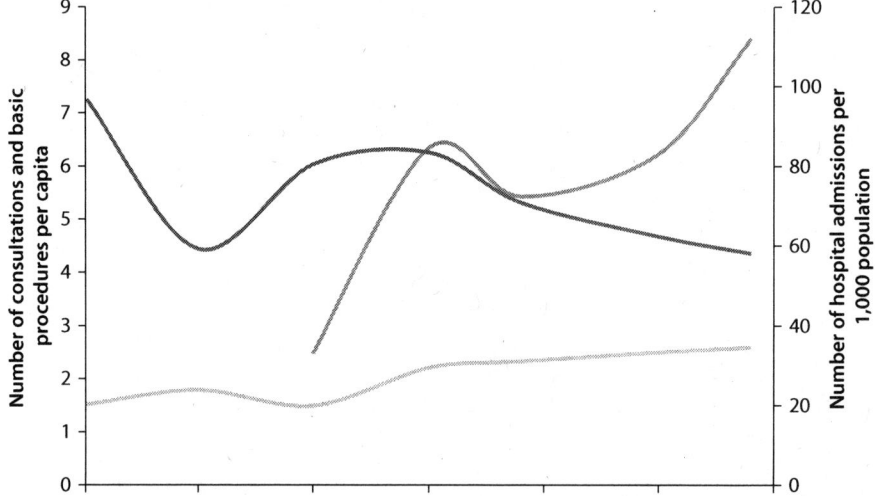

Sources: IBGE, AMS surveys (IBGE 2002, 2006, 2010); Ministry of Health DATASUS data.
Note: Changes in the list of procedures recorded in SUS information systems and their definition make comparisons over time imprecise; the figure for primary health care in 1990 is from IBGE AMS surveys and may not be strictly comparable to the figures for later years, which are from Ministry of Health data, but this is unlikely to change dramatically the general trend.

In the later years of this period, much of this increase was due to the rapid deployment of the Family Health Strategy (ESF). In contrast, the quantity of hospitalizations provided by the SUS or INAMPS remained stagnant at around 11.5 million, reaching a peak of 14.8 million in 1993. This translates into slightly declining hospital admission rates.

The composition of SUS service provision by type of provider also changed substantially, reflecting a change in the allocation of resources in favor of public providers and away from private contracted providers. This is especially apparent in the case of hospital care (figure 3.4). However, while hospitalizations in the SUS have been relatively stable, even falling between 1992 and 2009, hospitalizations in the private non-SUS sector have doubled, and by 2005 the private sector accounted for almost the same number of hospitalizations as the SUS. This raises important questions about whether constraints in SUS hospital capacity have resulted in rationing, with an overflow into the private sector, or whether other factors are at play.

Survey data corroborate administrative data on the volume and composition of services. For instance, the percentage of individuals who reported seeking some form of health care in the last two weeks increased nearly 30 percent between 1986 and 2008, from 11.3 to 14.4 percent. The type of services used by households also changed over time, with preventive visits and dental consultations accounting for a growing share of all visits to health care providers (figure 3.5). Moreover, the restructuring of health care provision and the strengthening of primary health care changed how Brazilians seek and use health care services. Up to the 1980s, hospitals were the preferred source of care for most Brazilians; 20 years later, more Brazilians use basic care units (and, to a lesser extent, private practice offices and clinics) as their main source of care (figure 3.6).

Figure 3.4 Hospital Admissions in Brazil, by Type of Provider, 1985–2009

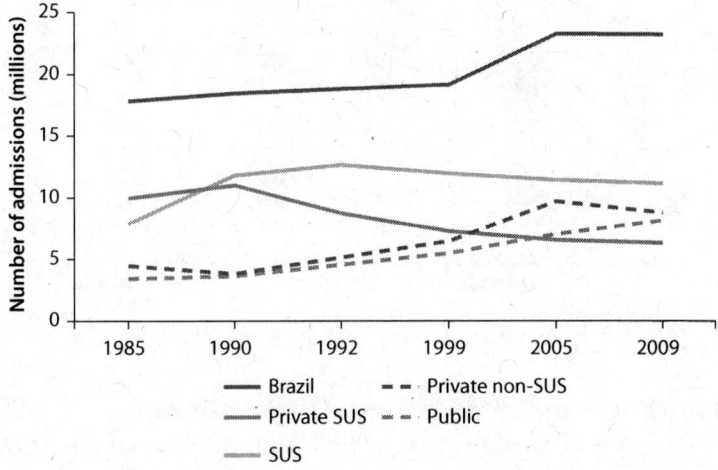

Sources: IBGE, AMS surveys (IBGE 2002, 2006, 2010); Ministry of Health DATASUS data.
Note: SUS = Sistema Único de Saúde. The line for Brazil includes public and private (SUS and non-SUS providers); the SUS line includes most admissions in public facilities and admissions in private facilities under SUS contract (private SUS).

Figure 3.5 Health Services Used by Households in Brazil, 1986 and 2008

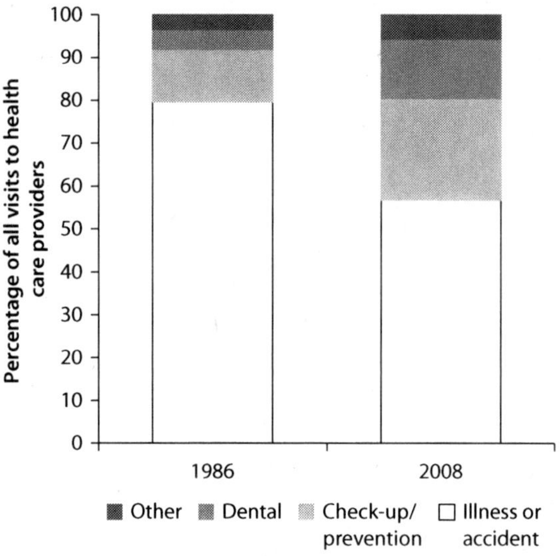

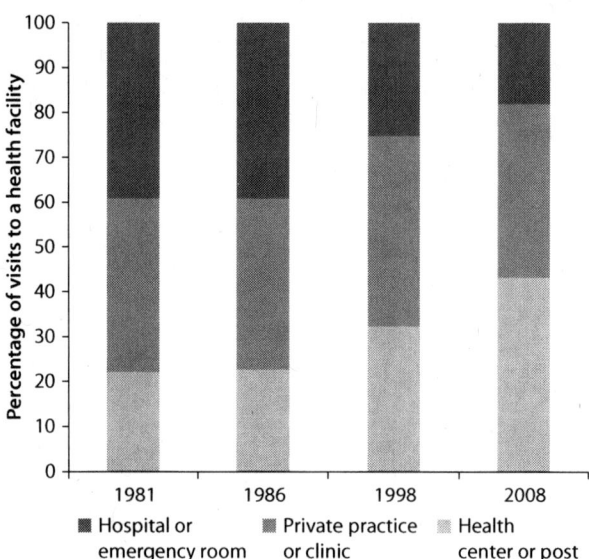

Source: Based on data from IBGE, PNAD for 1986 and 2008.

Figure 3.6 Source of Care in Brazil, by Type of Facility, 1981–2008

Source: Based on IBGE, PNAD for 2008.

Utilization Rates across States and Socioeconomic Groups

The gradual equalization of the availability of services across states, achieved by restructuring the hospital system and focusing the ESF rollout on the poorer states, has helped to reduce geographic disparities in utilization, although the picture is not entirely clear. By 2009, all states had achieved rates of at least 2.35

consultations per capita per year (figure 3.7). Increases in utilization were greater in low-income states, such that the relationship between average income and utilization was somewhat weaker (figure 3.8). In the case of hospitalizations, most states saw a reduction in admission rates (figure 3.7). Nonetheless, 90 percent of states achieved a hospital admission rate within the Ministry of Health (Ministério da Saúde) parameter of 7–9 percent per year (the exceptions are Alagoas, Amazonas, and Sergipe); the national average for 2008 was 9.0 percent. These rates are much lower than in Organisation for Economic Co-operation and Development (OECD) countries (6.8 percent for consultations and 15.8 percent for hospitalizations, respectively), but around or above those of most middle-income countries (2.5 and 5.5 percent, respectively, for Mexico) and significantly higher than those of China, Peru, and Thailand.[4] Although geographic disparities in utilization have declined somewhat, a significant income gradient remains in average utilization rates across states in Brazil (figure 3.8).

Moreover, notable disparities are still evident across income groups, with higher levels of utilization among high-income groups. For instance, household survey data indicate that utilization rates are around 50 percent higher for the top two deciles than for the bottom two (figure 3.9). The better off are also using SUS services at a much lower rate than those at the lower end of the income distribution.

Figure 3.7 SUS Consultations per Capita and Hospitalizations per 100 Persons in Brazil, by State, 1995 and 2008 (or 2009)

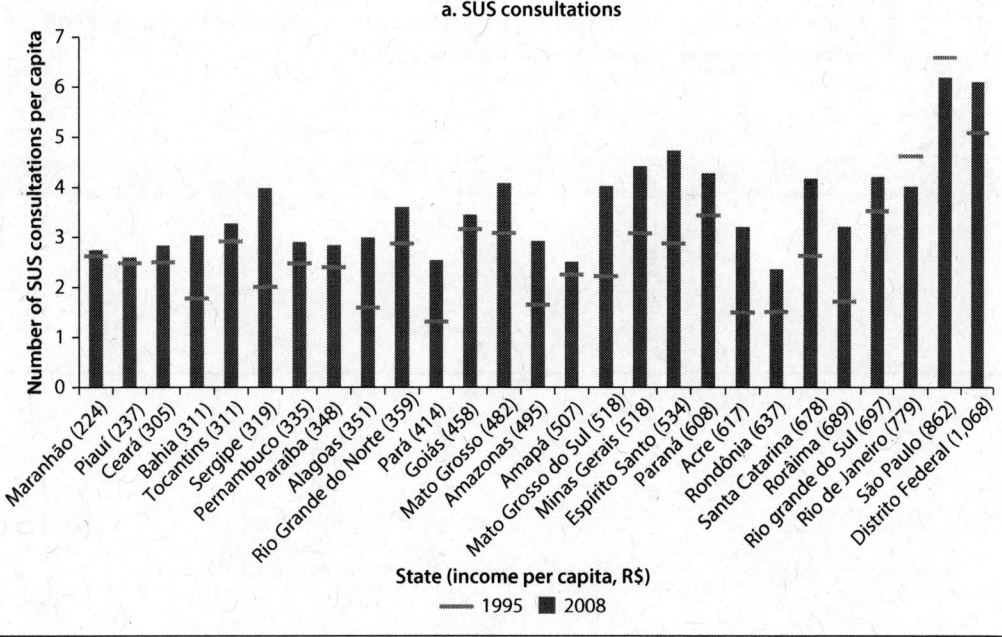

a. SUS consultations

State (income per capita, R$)

1995   2008

Figure 3.7   SUS Consultations per Capita and Hospitalizations per 100 Persons in Brazil, by State, 1995 and 2008 (or 2009) *(continued)*

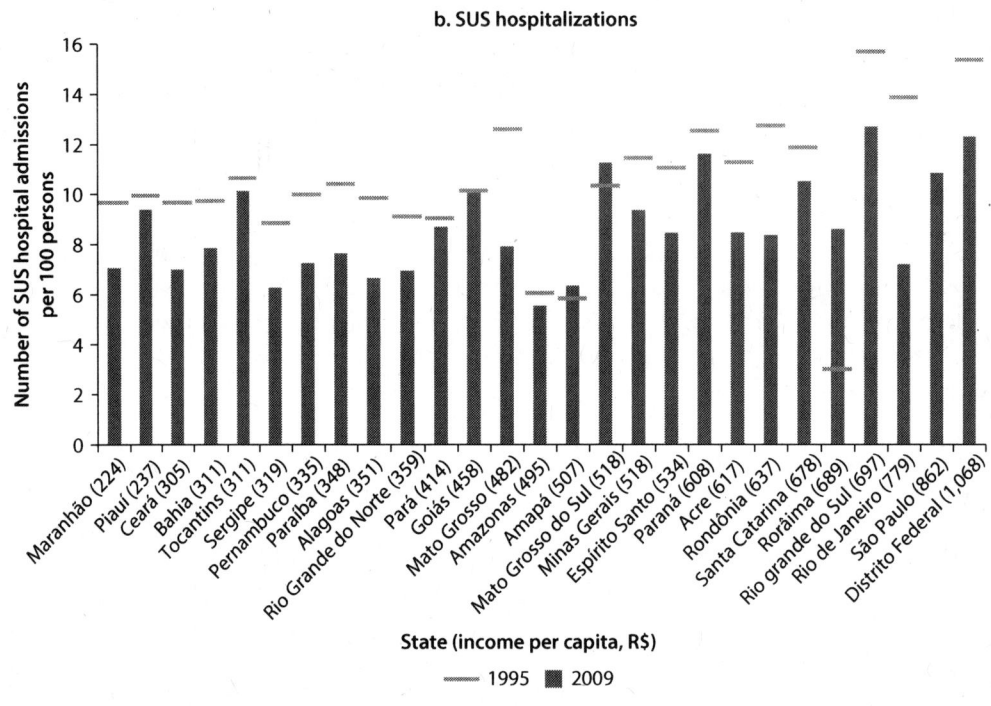

b. SUS hospitalizations

State (income per capita, R$)

―――― 1995 ■ 2009

Source: Based on Ministry of Health, DATASUS data.
Note: SUS = Sistema Único de Saúde. States are ranked by average income per capita (IPEAData).

Figure 3.8   SUS Consultations per Capita and Hospitalizations per 100 Persons in Brazil, by State Income per Capita, 1995 and 2008 (or 2009)

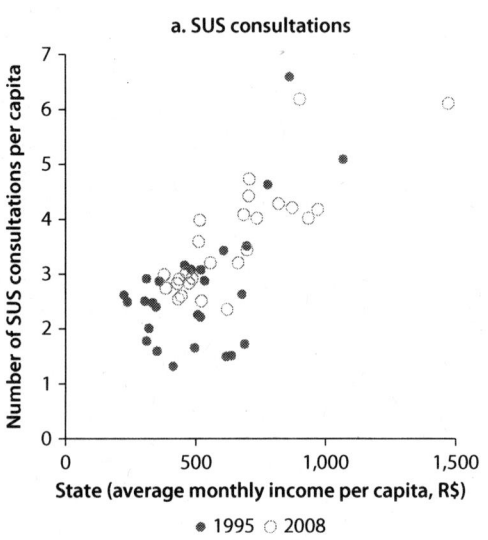

a. SUS consultations

State (average monthly income per capita, R$)

● 1995 ○ 2008

figure continues next page

Figure 3.8 SUS Consultations per Capita and Hospitalizations per 100 Persons in Brazil, by State Income per Capita, 1995 and 2008 (or 2009) *(continued)*

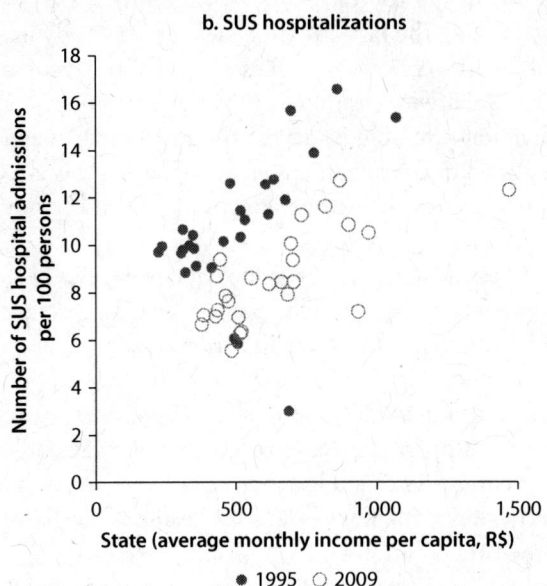

b. SUS hospitalizations

● 1995 ○ 2009

Sources: Based on Ministry of Health, DATASUS data; IPEAData from IBGE for state income levels.
Note: SUS = Sistema Único de Saúde.

Figure 3.9 Percentage of the Population Who Sought and Used Care in Brazil, by Income Decile, 1986 and 2008

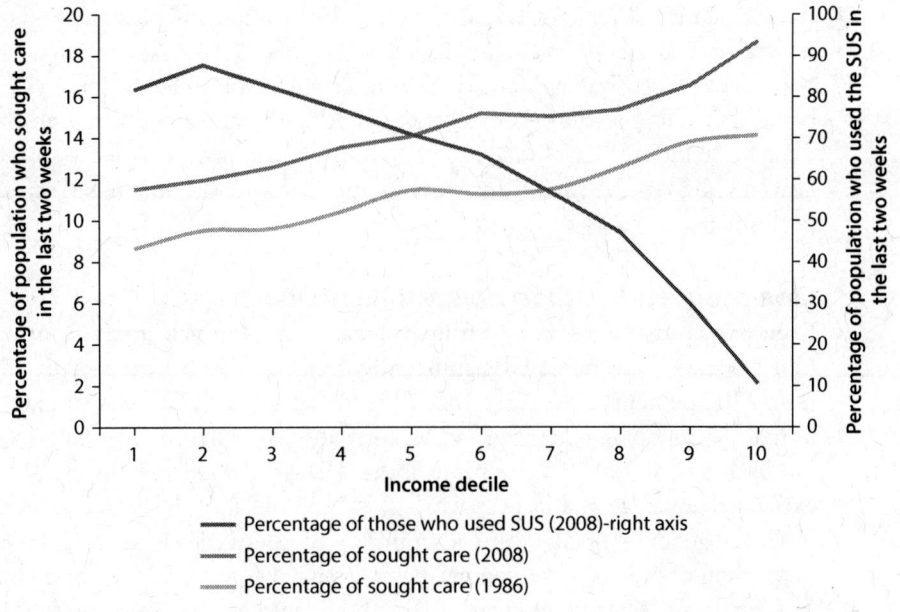

—— Percentage of those who used SUS (2008)-right axis
—— Percentage of sought care (2008)
—— Percentage of sought care (1986)

Source: IBGE, PNAD for 2008–09.
Note: SUS = Sistema Único de Saúde. Income decile is defined relative to mean household income per capita.

Are Health Care Needs Being Met?

Trends and patterns in the use of health services provide a good indication of realized access. As noted, the last 20 years have seen a steady increase in the use of many types of health services, as well as a reduction in geographic and socio-economic disparities. However, simple utilization rates do not shed much light on whether individuals are able to access the preventive, diagnostic, and curative services they need in a timely manner, even though this is a critical element in assessing progress toward improving access and achieving universal coverage.

One way to address this question is to look at coverage of health interventions with a clearly defined target group. This can be done, for instance, with maternal and child health interventions, such as immunizations, antenatal care, and hospital deliveries. Where data are available and the target population has been clearly defined, it is also possible to look at coverage rates for routine screening or disease management programs. As shown below, coverage of key maternal and child health interventions in Brazil has increased over the last couple of decades and is now nearly universal; fewer data are available on coverage of disease screening and other interventions.

Another approach is to look at self-reported unmet need. Household survey data in Brazil show a reduction in self-reported unmet need as well as a shift in the reasons reported for not using health services when needed. One of the limitations of self-reported problems with access is that questions tend to be concerned only with the use and nonuse of services. However, many care-seeking experiences involve multiple providers and services (general practice, specialist care, diagnostic services), with effective access depending not only on the availability of services, but also on the organization and coordination of care, referral arrangements, and so forth. Access is harder to assess in relation to these types of services, but is increasingly important as basic health care needs are being met and the burden of chronic conditions increases. Although limited, available evidence from Brazil points to important weaknesses in the system and also highlights the need for more systematic data on these aspects of performance.

Coverage of Key Health Services and Interventions

Even prior to the extension of primary health care through the ESF, immunization coverage had increased significantly, from around 50 percent in 1980 to nearly 100 percent in the early 2000s (figure 3.10). This trend was similar to that in many developing countries and somewhat weaker than in some middle- and low-income countries; for example, India, Malaysia, Mexico, Peru, and Thailand expanded coverage at a faster pace.

Coverage of antenatal care also improved. Between 1996 and 2006, the proportion of pregnant women having no prenatal consultation dropped from 26 to 1.3 percent (Ministry of Health 2010b) the mean number of consultations rose from 1.2 to 6.2, and the share of women with at least four visits during pregnancy

Figure 3.10 Immunization Coverage in Brazil and Other Developing Countries, 1980–2009

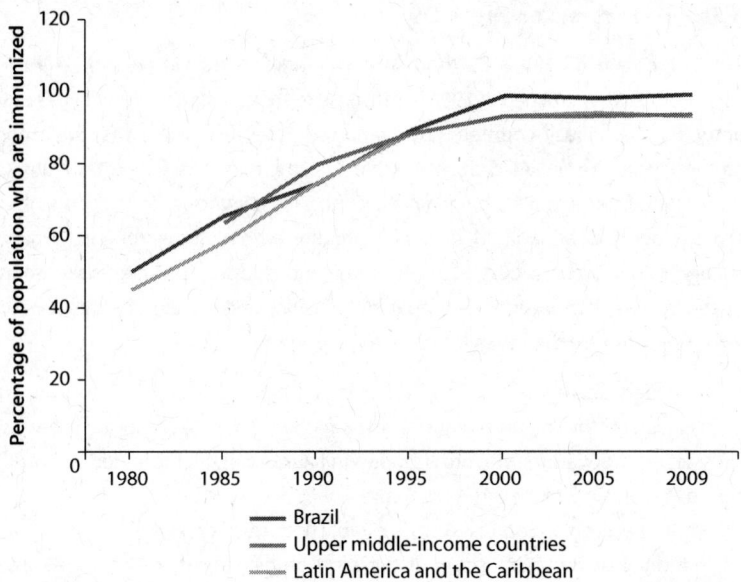

Sources: Ministry of Health and World Bank data.

increased from 76 to 89 percent, which was higher than that in other countries with available data.

At the other end of the spectrum, the Program on HIV/AIDS (human immunodeficiency virus/acquired immunodeficiency syndrome) has been very successful and one of the few programs to offer nearly universal access to AIDS medications and treatment (box 3.1). The program's success was also due to a strong health education initiative conducted through the media, which induced significant change in health and sexual behavior.

Trends and Patterns in the Use and Nonuse of Services

Another indicator of access is the proportion of people reporting that they did not seek health services when they perceived a need for care.[5] While there has been no clear trend in the nonuse of services for individuals who reported an episode of illness over the last decade, there has been an important shift in the relative importance of the reasons for not seeking care. In particular, the share of households reporting lack of money (for services or transportation) as a reason for not using services declined over the last two decades, in particular among households at the lower end of the income distribution (figure 3.11). Similarly, the expansion of infrastructure and staffing has translated into improved availability of services, with fewer households reporting access or transportation as a reason for not seeking care.

Meanwhile, facility-related reasons (lack of or unfriendly staff, inadequate scheduling, long waiting times) have increased, becoming the chief reasons for

Box 3.1 Brazil's Program on HIV/AIDS

The Brazilian Program on HIV/AIDS (human immunodeficiency virus/acquired immunodeficiency syndrome) was launched in 1986 in response to the rapid expansion of the epidemic in the country. By then, Brazil counted 1,537 reported cases, a number that was more than doubling every year. The HIV/AIDS policy ultimately combined several key strategies: (a) mass media information campaigns, (b) wide availability of diagnosis, (c) free distribution of antiretroviral drugs to all patients, (d) close collaboration with nongovernmental organizations and patients' rights organizations, (e) focus on and support for high-risk groups, and (f) negotiations with pharmaceutical companies to reduce prices under the threat of breaking patents. The following are the key milestones of the program:

- *1984.* The Health Secretariat of São Paulo establishes the first AIDS control program; Montagnier isolates the retrovirus causing the infection: 220 cases reported (prevalence).
- *1985.* The first nongovernmental organization in Latin America is founded in Brazil (Grupo de Apoio à Prevenção à AIDS, GAPA): 678 cases.
- *1986.* The national Program on HIV/AIDS is established: 1,537 cases.
- *1988.* The federal government starts distributing drugs against opportunistic infections: 6,029 cases.
- *1991.* The Ministry of Health starts distributing free antiretroviral drugs: 18,487 cases.
- *1992.* The Ministry of Health launches a large education campaign and begins to reimburse treatment under the SUS: 25,186 cases.
- *1994.* A World Bank support project is initiated: 38,015 cases.
- *1996.* The Program on HIV/AIDS launches the first national consensus for AIDS treatment; the free distribution of antiretroviral drugs is established by law: 56,605 cases.
- *1998.* Treatment coverage is mandated for private insurers; the Ministry of Health begins to distribute 11 drugs: 91,916 cases.
- *2001.* Brazil threatens to break patents and negotiates a significant reduction in the price of antiretroviral drugs: 139,573 cases.
- *2007.* Survival rates improve significantly; the Ministry of Health establishes a database on violations of HIV/AIDS patients' rights: 474,273 cases since 1980.
- *2008.* Brazil invests US$10 million in a factory producing antiretroviral drugs in Mozambique.

The program managed to change sexual behavior through information campaigns, achieved nearly universal free treatment, was a leader in negotiating significant reductions in drug prices, and ultimately controlled expansion of the epidemic and reduced mortality from HIV/AIDS (mortality peaked in 1995, reaching 12.2 deaths out of 100,000 population and then dropped to half by 1998).

Source: Ministry of Health, Departamento de DST, AIDS e Hepatites Virais website (http://www.aids.gov.br).

not seeking care. These data strongly suggest that access to services has improved, but that the problems with quality and responsiveness of services have worsened (or expectations have risen).[6] This is also apparent from the increase in the share of households that report seeking care but not being able to access it (figure 3.12).

Figure 3.11 Reasons Given for Not Seeking Care in Brazil, by Income Decile, 1986 and 2008

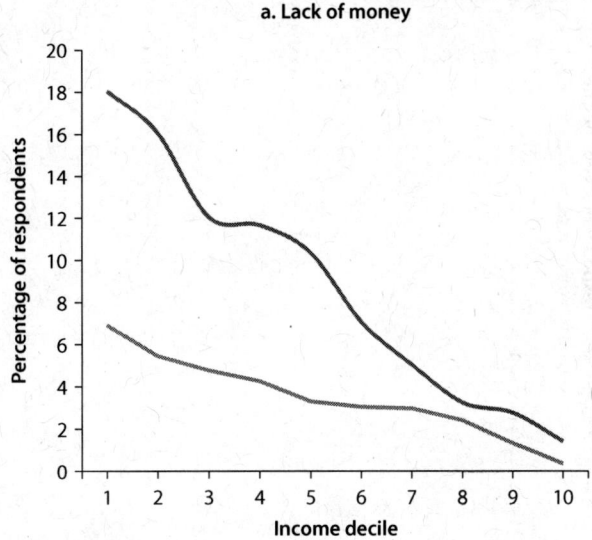

a. Lack of money

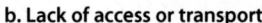

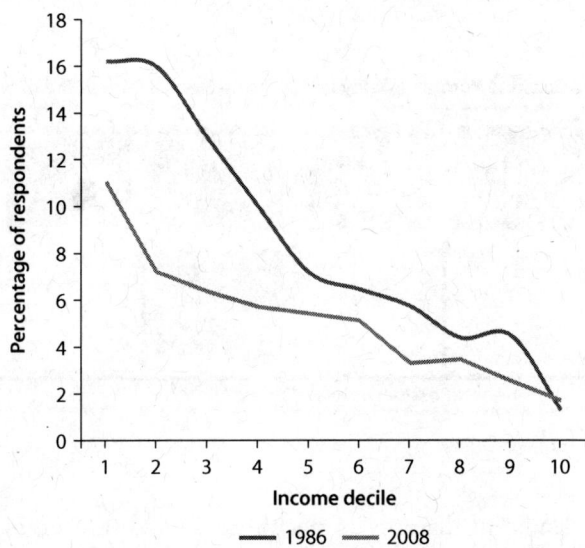

b. Lack of access or transport

1986 ——— 2008

Source: IBGE, PNAD for 1986 and 2008.

Access to Specialist Care and Waiting Times

Data from household or patient surveys on the nonuse of services can provide important insights into access problems. In many cases, such data refer to primary contacts in the event of illness or need (as perceived by the respondent). Yet, as illustrated in figure 3.13, many health needs require services and clinical decisions from multiple providers, and problems with access and delays in receiving care can arise at various points in this process.

Figure 3.12 Share of Persons Reporting That They Sought Care but Did Not Receive It in Brazil, by Income Decile, 1986 and 2008

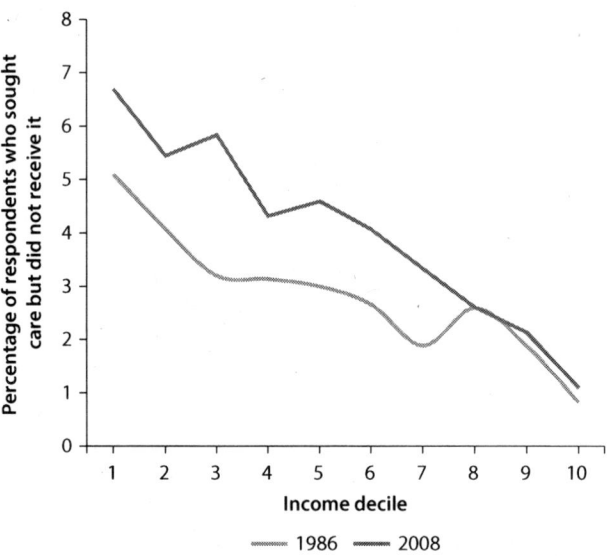

Source: IBGE, PNAD for 1986 and 2008.

Figure 3.13 Patterns of Care and Possible Points of Delay in Accessing Health Care in Brazil

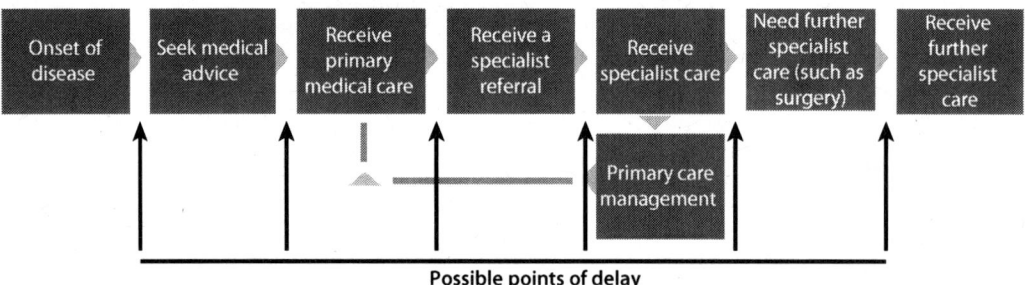

Source: Authors

Given the significant diversity of health needs and the complex pattern of health care provided to patients, access problems along this chain are hard to capture in simple indicators. One common approach is to assess the performance of health systems through data on waiting times, typically for elective procedures. Indeed, waiting times are one of the most important health system problems in many OECD countries (OECD 2003). While there is no established consensus on what represents an "excessive" waiting time, many countries have established targets for maximum waiting times, on the grounds that longer waiting times are unpopular and can lead to adverse consequences (such as deterioration in the condition, anxiety, increase in the cost of the procedure, and loss of income from work).

There is ample evidence that long waiting times are a source of considerable frustration among users of the SUS. However, systematic data are scarce on how long patients are waiting for specialist assessments and care. A recent study of cancer care by the Federal Audit Tribunal (Tribunal de Contas da União, TCU 2011) represents an important effort to compile data on delays in diagnosis and treatment that illustrate broader challenges in the health system. Cancer is now the second most important cause of mortality in Brazil, and demand for both diagnostic and treatment services is increasing rapidly. Using administrative data on payments for high-complexity procedures from 2010, the study found that, as a result of problems accessing diagnostic procedures and specialist care, 60 percent of cancer patients were diagnosed at a very late stage (stage three or four), reducing the prospects of effective treatment and survival.[7] There are no directly comparable data from multicountry studies, but in the United States, only 7 percent of cancer patients were diagnosed at stage three or four according to a recent study (Legorreta *et al.* 2004).

The problem of late diagnosis is compounded by delays in accessing treatment. The report uses both administrative data on authorized payments for radiation and chemotherapy and hospital cancer registries to assess the delay from diagnosis to treatment. Payment data indicate that median waiting time for chemotherapy was 76.3 days in 2010, with only 35.6 percent of patients receiving treatment within 30 days of diagnosis. In the case of radiation therapy, the corresponding figures were 113.4 days and 15.9 percent of patients.[8] There are no national guidelines or targets against which to assess these numbers. However, as a point of comparison, the report notes that in Canada and the United Kingdom most patients receive treatment within 30 days (88 and 99 percent, respectively), with a median waiting time ranging from 5 to 25 days depending on the type of treatment.

The report notes that delays in diagnosis and treatment are inconsistent with the goals established in Law 8.080 and the National Cancer Policy (Portaria GM/MS 2.439/2005). Several factors contribute to the problem, including a lack of capacity in the system, insufficient staff with qualifications in relevant specialties (such as pathologists), weaknesses in the referral and counterreferral systems, and payment rates that do not always match the costs of services.[9] More and better data are needed on waiting times and outcomes (such as survival rates).

Another effort to assess unmet need is a recent study focusing on the demand for specialist, diagnostic, and surgical procedures in Rio Grande do Sul (CNM 2011). The study collected data on all referrals for which the service had not yet been provided to the patient and found that, for the state as a whole, with a population of 10.6 million people, there was an unmet need of nearly 500,000 consultations or procedures.[10] Specialist consultations (orthopedic and opthalmology were the most important) accounted for more than half of these, while diagnostic procedures accounted for 30 percent. In the case of hospital admissions, nearly all of the unmet need was for psychiatric care. These problems are attributed to a lack of physical capacity, inadequate financing by the state, and weaknesses in the referral and counter-referral systems.

Data on waiting lists and access to specialist care are limited in Brazil. Nonetheless, many patients clearly have difficulty navigating the health system, which explains the comparatively high levels of dissatisfaction with the SUS.

The Quality Dimension: A Missing Piece of the Puzzle?

Discussions of coverage tend to focus on access to and cost of services for different groups. However, this concept of "coverage" does not adequately capture quality and the extent to which improvements in coverage of health services translate into better health outcomes. In other words, it is not only access to services that matters for realizing potential health gains, but also the extent to which those services are appropriate and well delivered.[11]

Although enhanced effectiveness was an important goal, the SUS reform did not focus explicitly on quality. This may be due to the fact that the quality of health services is inherently difficult to measure. Indeed, the quality of services in the Brazilian health system has only recently been reported or monitored and even then only partially. While long-term comparisons are difficult to make, quality has been a long-standing concern. For instance, a report from 1994 found that, in the early 1990s, little systematic information or rigorous assessment of the quality of care was available, and a huge contrast existed between world-class quality in complex services, such as cardiac surgery and transplants, and generally inadequate quality in the most-used basic services, such as maternal and child care (World Bank 1994). Among other things, the report noted (a) inappropriate patterns of staffing and work; (b) inadequate patterns of drug prescription and use, with few facilities using a list of essential or standardized drugs; (c) high rates of Cesarean sections; (d) lack of standard treatment protocols; (e) high infection rates among surgical procedures and inpatient care in general (6.5–15 percent) and high mortality rates (13.9 percent in private hospitals under contract with INAMPS and 6.7 percent in public hospitals in Rio de Janeiro); (f) limited use of quality assurance programs; and (g) weak channels for reporting malpractice or consumer dissatisfaction.

Almost 15 years later, in their review of the hospital sector, La Forgia and Couttolenc (2008) found that progress had been slow and limited, in spite of the multiplication of quality assurance initiatives.[12] The study found several frequent quality issues that can be grouped into the following: errors or delays in diagnosis; failure to follow recommended procedures; failure to carry out operations and examinations using appropriate procedures; failure to select and administer treatments properly; mistakes in dosage or method of using or administering drugs; unnecessary delays in providing treatment or sharing test results; use of incorrect or inappropriate treatment; failure to use recommended prophylactic treatments; lack of a monitoring, revision, and control system; problems with availability and use of equipment; and lack of a staff training system (La Forgia and Couttolenc 2008).

Similar concerns have also been raised by other studies. For instance, a 2003 survey of more than 1,000 public and private hospitals in São Paulo State found that 52.5 percent—47.6 percent of public and 53.9 percent of private hospitals—did not comply with minimum requirements for licensing by state and national standards (CREMESP 2004) and that two-thirds had incomplete medical records. The Ministry of Health's Program for Evaluation of Health Services (Programa Nacional de Avaliação de Serviços de Saúde), in its 2005 report, found that, of the 6,030 SUS-funded hospitals surveyed, 40 percent did not respond and 37 percent were not compliant; among those that were rated, only 16 percent were deemed as providing good or superior quality of care, while 37 percent were seen as providing unacceptable or very unacceptable quality (Ministry of Health 2006). Clearly, quality concerns are related to weak design or implementation of regulatory and quality assurance systems, but provider payment arrangements and patient expectations also come into play. This is evident, for example, in the very high rates of Cesarean sections in Brazil (box 3.2).

But there are also indications of improvements. For instance, two recent studies used the Primary Care Assessment Tool of the Ministry of Health (2010a) to assess the quality of the ESF relative to the traditional approach to providing facility-based primary health care services and found that in all of the quality-related functions considered, the ESF was significantly superior to the traditional approach (Macinko 2011; Macinko, Almeida, and de Sá 2007; figure 3.14).

Other studies have focused on hospitalization for conditions that can be managed effectively in a primary care setting (with high hospital admission rates for these conditions indicating poor quality of primary care). The proportion of admissions for conditions sensitive to primary care was estimated in the early 2000s at 27 percent in Minas Gerais (SES-MG 2005) and at 30 percent in Brazil as a whole (La Forgia and Couttolenc 2008). However, during 1999–2007 hospitalizations for chronic diseases that are sensitive to outpatient care (cardiovascular disease, stroke, and asthma) fell at a rate greater than hospitalizations for other reasons. Moreover, the ESF had a lower proportion of avoidable admissions (Macinko 2011), as illustrated in figure 3.15. Similarly, a study by Dourado et al. (2011) looking at national, regional, and state-level data found that greater ESF coverage at the state level was associated with lower hospital admissions for conditions sensitive to primary health care, after controlling for confounding variables.

Health System Efficiency

The concept of efficiency is concerned with the relationship between inputs and outcomes or outputs. At the broadest level, an efficient health system is one that produces the greatest improvement for a given level of spending. Given the variegated influences on health outcomes, efficiency is difficult to determine at this high level. For these reasons, assessments of efficiency tend to focus on specific links in the chain from spending to outcomes, including the extent to which resources are allocated appropriately across programs or

Box 3.2 Cesarean Sections in Brazil

The proportion of Cesarean sections in Brazil has been among the highest in the world for many years and now averages 43 percent nationally. It has been increasing in all regions since the 1970s: from 15 percent in the early 1970s to 30–35 percent in the 1980s, 40 percent in the late 1990s, and 49 percent in 2008 (Victora *et al.* 2011). However, SUS (Sistema Único de Saúde) rates remain much higher in the rich states of the southeastern and southern regions (33–35 percent) than in the northern and northeastern regions (28 percent in 2007). The mean rate for Brazil is higher than in any other country and twice the 22 percent average for high-income countries (WHO 2008); it is much higher than the upper limit recommended by the World Health Organization (15 percent). Cesarean sections may be more convenient for physicians and many mothers, but they also carry increased risks for women and newborns.

The SUS, which is responsible for about 80 percent of deliveries, has been moderately successful at curbing the trend within its system, through changes in payment levels in the early 1980s and other policies in the 1990s; the rate would probably be much higher if the SUS had not implemented policies to reduce it.[13] The rate is much higher in the private sector (covered by health insurance plans), at more than 80 percent, than in the SUS (IBGE 2009). But the effects of SUS policies have been short-lived, as apparent in figure B3.2.1. Particularly worrisome is the 44 percent increase in the SUS rate since 2000 (32 percent increase in the private sector rate).

Figure B3.2.1 Rates of Cesarean Section for Brazil as a Whole and for INAMPS/SUS, 1970–2009

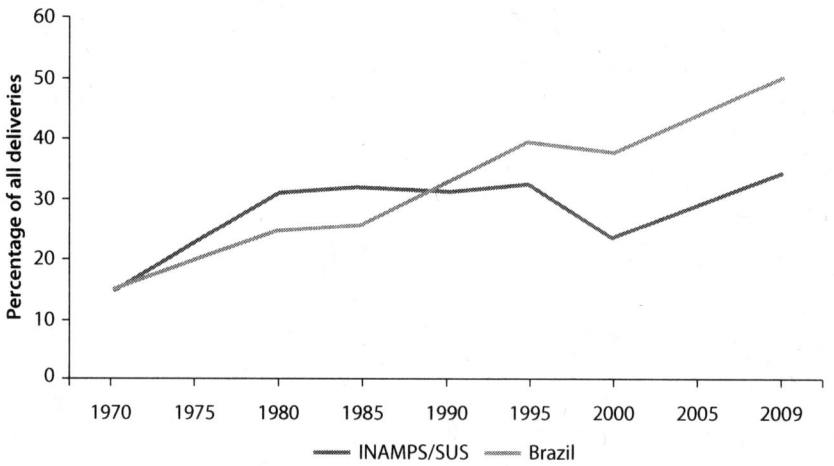

Sources: Ministry of Health data; Ministry of Health, SVS 2011; ANS 2011.
Note: INAMPS = Instituto Nacional de Assistência Médica da Previdência Social, SUS = Sistema Único de Saúde.

Figure 3.14 Quality of Care in the ESF and the Traditional Primary Health Care System in Petropolis, Brazil, 2003

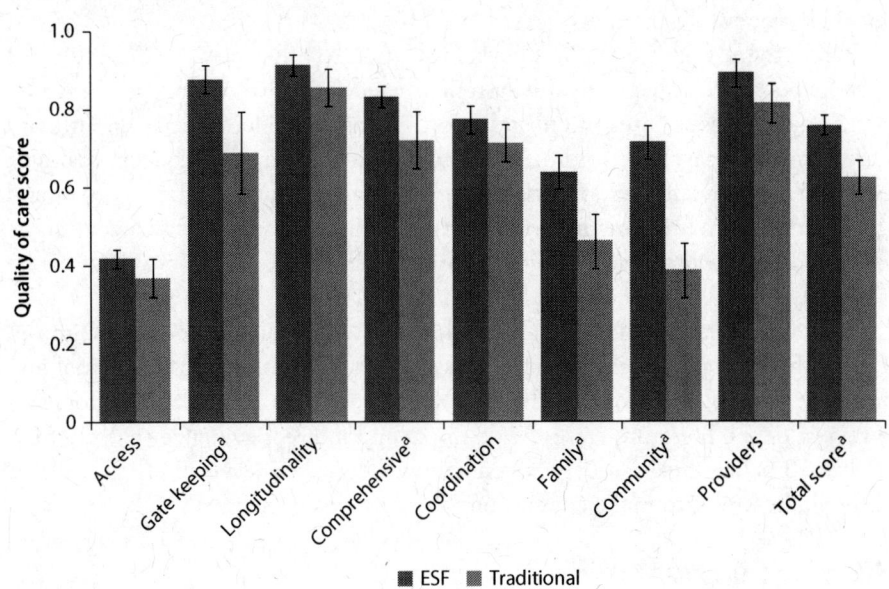

Source: Macinko, Almeida, and de Sá 2007.
a. Difference between reformed (ESF) and traditional clinics is statistically significant at less than 5 percent.

Figure 3.15 Potentially Avoidable Hospital Admissions for Chronic Diseases and ESF Coverage in Brazil, 1997–2007

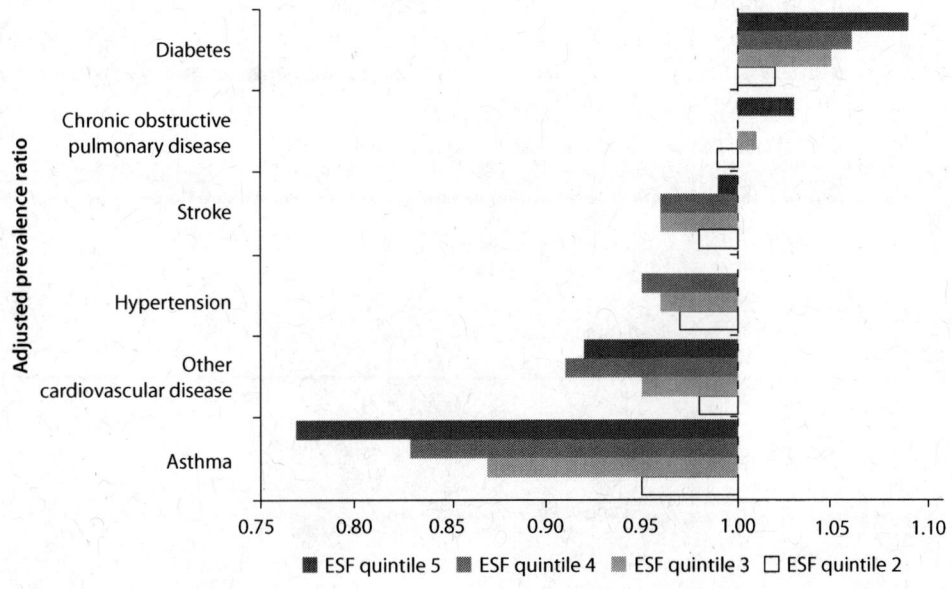

Source: Macinko 2011.
Note: ESF (Family Health Strategy) quintiles are based on a ranking of municipalities by level of ESF coverage, with quintile 1 being the municipalities with the lowest level of coverage and Q5 being the municipalities with the highest.

interventions (allocative efficiency) and the extent to which the greatest volume and quality of health services are produced for the available inputs (technical efficiency).

While there were no explicit goals in relation to efficiency, the SUS reforms were expected to enhance health system efficiency through a range of measures, including increased integration and coordination, enhanced focus on primary care, provider payment reform, and stronger governance and accountability. Many of these specific reforms, particularly in the areas of provider payment and governance, were implemented only partially; although gains in efficiency can be expected due to the strengthening of primary care, these gains are likely to be relatively small.

Few indicators of efficiency are available for an extended period of time in Brazil's health care system. The few studies on the issue are cross-sectional and focus on particular aspects of efficiency. However, some available indicators and a review of the literature can provide direct and indirect evidence that the SUS and the Brazilian health sector in general operate at low levels of efficiency. It is difficult, however, to make conclusions about trends over time.

Allocative Efficiency

Few studies have been conducted of allocative efficiency in the Brazilian health system. However, government spending has been reallocated toward primary care, with the share allocated to basic care increasing from 10 percent in the 1970s to around 20 percent in 2010, while medium- and high-complexity care continues to account for the largest share of spending. Nonetheless, the changes in resource allocation are bringing Brazil more in line with OECD countries, where inpatient, including long-term, care accounts for 41 percent of health expenditure, ranging between 34 and 52 percent, and outpatient, including primary and secondary, care accounts for 31 percent, ranging between 23 and 46 percent (figure 3.16).[14]

Figure 3.16 Distribution of Health Spending in OECD Countries, 2007

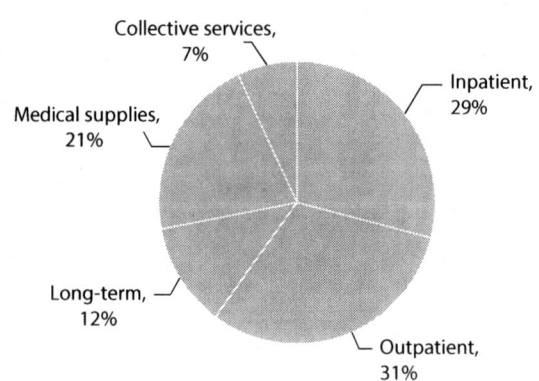

Source: OECD 2011.
Note: OECD = Organisation for Economic Co-operation and Development.

Medical Technology and Allocative Efficiency at the Facility Level

Brazil is an avid adopter of medical technologies. However, a substantial proportion of high-complexity equipment is adopted without considering its implications for the cost, quality, and effectiveness of care. In 2002, Brazil as a whole had a density for computerized tomography (CT) and magnetic resonance imaging (MRI) scanners higher than that of the lowest quartile of OECD countries, which includes countries from Eastern Europe, and close to that of a group of five rich countries that are relatively low users of medical technology and have established systems to regulate the adoption of new technology (Australia, Canada, France, the Netherlands, and the United Kingdom; figure 3.17).

The availability of equipment is much lower in the SUS than in Brazil as a whole, because the larger part is offered by the private (not-for-SUS) sector, where supply is much higher than in most OECD countries. In addition, the allocation of high-cost medical equipment in Brazil is largely irrational and inefficient: an analysis of density by municipality in 2002 revealed that, of the 100 municipalities with the highest density, 70 percent had fewer than 30,000 inhabitants and had densities more than 10 times higher than among OECD countries (Couttolenc, Dias, and Nicolella 2004). This means that a substantial proportion of high-cost equipment is installed in municipalities that have neither the size nor the role (within the health system) to host them.

However, the supply of diagnostic equipment tends to generate demand for it, at a high cost to the health system. SUS supply is in line with Ministry of Health standards but relatively high in comparison to that of most upper-middle-income countries (typically the lowest quartile of OECD countries). No established system for regulating and organizing the adoption and supply of medical technology is yet in place, although partial initiatives have been undertaken by the Ministry of Health, such as the establishment of a specific department and financing of some studies on the issue.

Another indicator of the supply and use of technical inputs is the mean number of diagnostic tests per medical consultation. This number increased 80 percent between 1995 and 2008, from 0.1 to 0.18 (Ministry of Health, DATASUS data). However, some studies indicate that up to 60 percent of diagnostic tests are unwarranted and useless: they reveal little that could not be revealed by a simple examination of the patient and add little value to diagnosis and treatment (Santos 2006). This also reflects the low use of treatment guidelines in Brazil.

Hospital Efficiency

Efficiency in hospital care can be measured in several ways, such as bed occupancy rate, staff productivity, and use of hospital infrastructure. Most Brazilian hospitals operate at a very low level of efficiency. Using data envelopment analysis for a sample of 428 hospitals, La Forgia and Couttolenc (2008) found that the average score for technical efficiency in 2002 was 0.34 on a scale of 0 of 1, which means that the average hospital could produce three times more output if it were as efficient as the most efficient hospital in the sample. Public

Figure 3.17 Density of Technology Use in Brazil and OECD Countries, 1985–2009

a. CT scanners

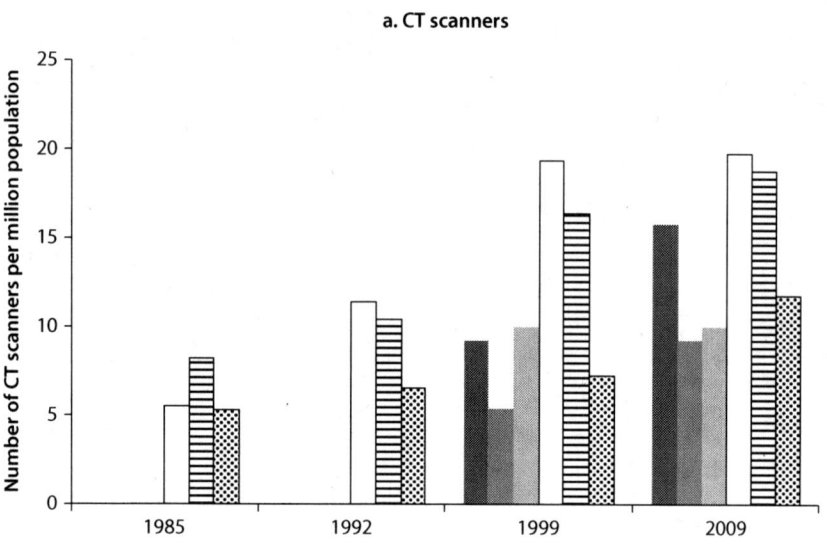

b. MRIs

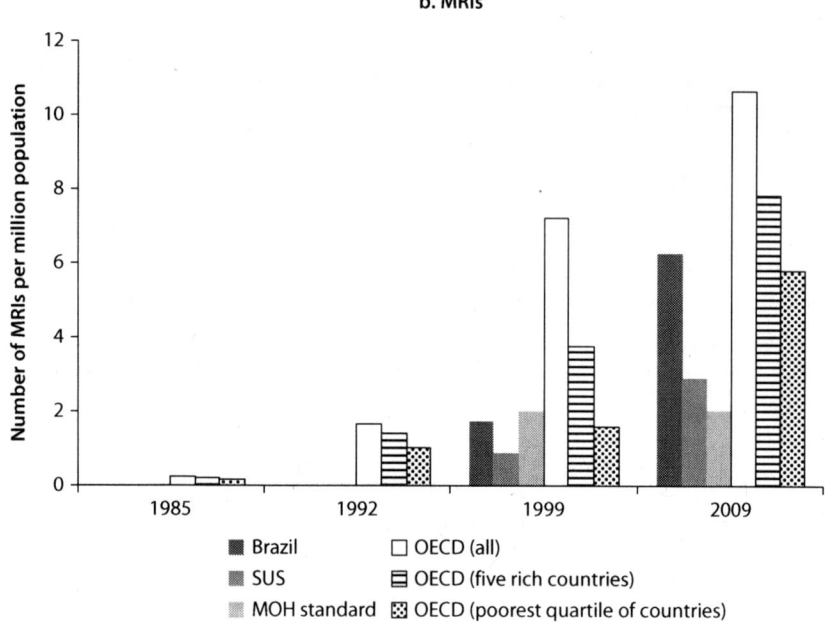

Sources: Couttolenc, Dias, and Nicolella 2004, with data from AMS surveys (IBGE 2002, 2006, 2010); (OECD 2011) IBGE 2009.
Note: CT = computerized tomography, MOH = Ministry of Health, MRI = magnetic resonance imaging, OECD = Organisation for Economic Co-operation and Development, SUS = Sistema Único de Saúde.

hospitals were less efficient than private ones (mean score of 0.29 and 0.39, respectively), but both were, on average, quite inefficient. The main factors contributing to inefficiency were small scale of operations, high use of human resources, and low use of installed capacity and technical resources. The governance model and payment mechanisms also affected efficiency.

Most Brazilian hospitals are too small to operate efficiently: 65 percent have fewer than 50 beds, and only 13 percent have 100 beds or more, while the international literature and La Forgia and Couttolenc (2008) have found that efficient hospitals tend to be have more than 200 beds. The large number of small hospitals in Brazil is to some extent the result of a deliberate SUS policy to extend access to hospital care in smaller cities by building a large number of small municipal hospitals. Between 1985 and 1999, some 1,200 new public hospitals were built—mostly municipal—and the average size dropped from 94 to 55 beds (IBGE 2002, 2006, 2010).

The mean bed occupancy rate in Brazil is very low and an important source of inefficiency and waste. La Forgia and Couttolenc (2008) found that the bed occupancy rate among SUS hospitals was 37 percent for acute care hospitals and 45 percent for all hospitals (compared with the level recommended by the Ministry of Health of 75–85 percent and international averages of around 70–75 percent). Many hospitals had a bed occupancy rate below 25 percent. As shown in figure 3.18, low bed occupancy rates have been an issue in SUS hospitals for many years, although they improved gradually in the 2000s.

Hospital technical resources are also underutilized. For instance, the mean number of surgeries performed per operating theater in Brazil was 0.66 per working day (La Forgia and Couttolenc 2008); this means that operating rooms

Figure 3.18 Bed Occupancy Rate in SUS Hospitals in Brazil, 1992–2010

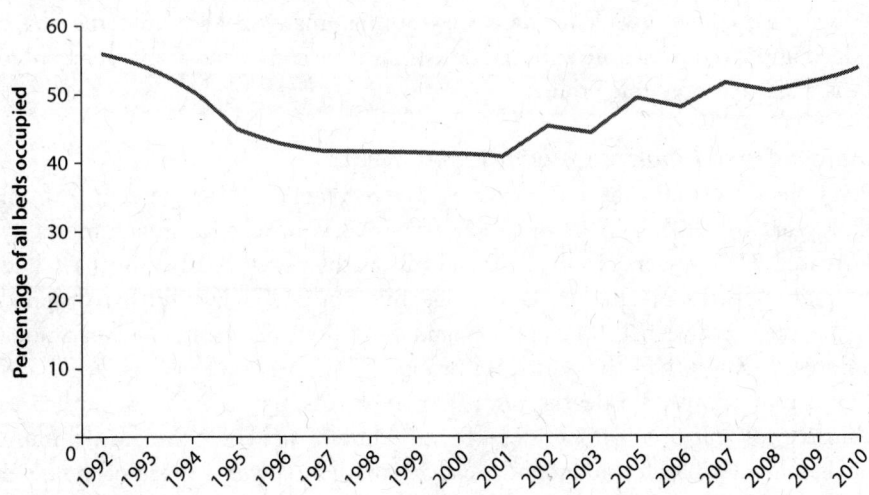

Source: Ministry of Health, DATASUS data.
Note: SUS = Sistema Único de Saúde. Figure is for all SUS hospitals, both acute and chronic care; the rate for acute care hospitals is about 10 percentage points lower.

in the typical Brazilian hospital are not used 85 percent of the time. In fact, such low use of available infrastructure and resources hides two quite different realities: a small number of large referral hospitals are heavily used, as reflected in long lines and crowded rooms and corridors, while most small hospitals are hardly used at all. Since most Brazilians tend to bypass small local hospitals and seek care at large regional facilities, the policy to extend access through a large network of small hospitals has proved ineffective and costly.

It is unclear whether the bed occupancy rate was affected by the expansion and strengthening of primary health care in the mid-1990s and the ceiling defined for inpatient admissions, since at the same time some 500 new—mostly small—hospitals were built. Also, part of hospitals' inefficiency is a result of ineffective primary care and poor referral mechanisms. For instance, two studies estimated the proportion of hospital admissions for conditions sensitive to outpatient care within the SUS at close to 30 percent; in comparison, studies in Spain and the United States found much lower proportions (8–18 and 13–16 percent, respectively).[15] The use of hospital infrastructure for unneeded admissions is clearly related to the absence of functioning, effective health care networks.

Has the Health System Improved Health Outcomes?

Ensuring broad-based access to effective health services was a key concern of the SUS reforms. However, as noted in chapter 1, the ultimate goal of health systems is to improve the level and distribution of health outcomes, to ensure that financing of health care is affordable and equitable, and to achieve high levels of responsiveness and satisfaction.

While the SUS founding legislation did not define any specific target for health outcomes, the reforms were expected to improve health outcomes and reduce inequalities. Available data suggest that many health outcomes have indeed improved over time and that outcomes have converged across geographic areas and socioeconomic groups.

Improved Health Outcomes, with Some Caveats

First, life expectancy at birth increased 9.8 years or 15.5 percent,[16] from 63.3 years in 1985 to 73.1 in 2009 (figure 3.19). Second, infant mortality decreased 71.3 percent, from 60.3 to 17.3 deaths per 1,000 live births. Child mortality (deaths of children under age five per 1,000 live births) dropped 57.6 percent between 1990 and 2008, and mortality from acute diarrhea among children younger than five years old dropped 71.5 percent between 1990 and 2007 (from 12.3 to 3.5 deaths per 1,000 live births; figure 3.20). According to Ministry of Health projections, Brazil should achieve the Millennium Development Goals for infant and child mortality three years ahead of the 2015 deadline (Ministry of Health 2010b).

Comparing the progress in outcome indicators with that of other countries sheds additional light on the issue. Since 1985, life expectancy and infant

Figure 3.19 Long-Term Trends in Life Expectancy and Infant Mortality in Brazil, 1960–2009

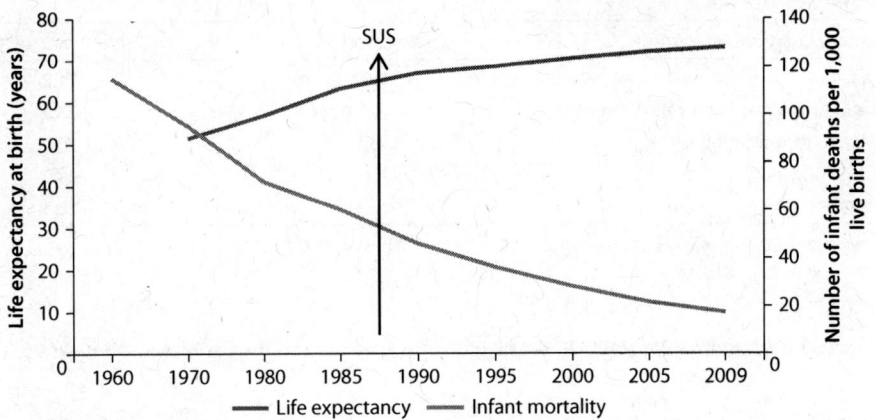

Sources: IBGE 2009 Ministry of Health, SUS 2011.
Note: SUS = Sistema Único de Saúde.

Figure 3.20 Child Mortality and Mortality by Acute Diarrhea among Children Younger Than Five Years Old in Brazil, 1990–2008

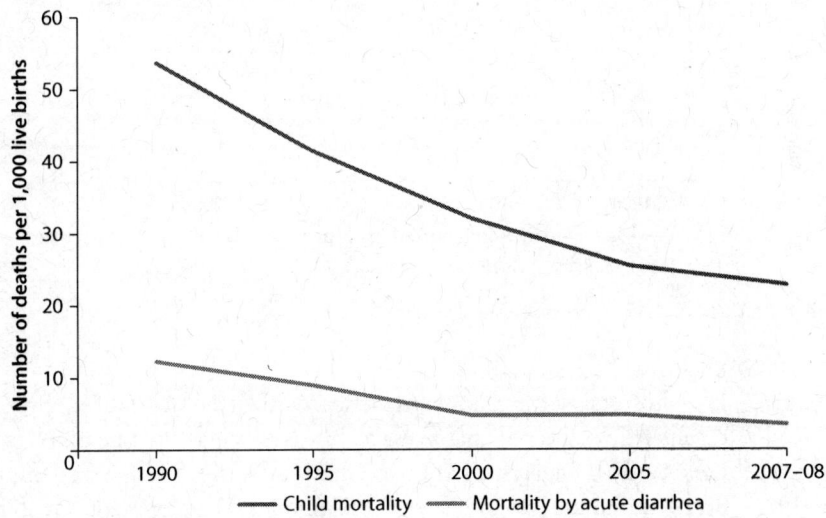

Sources: Ministry of Health data (Ministry of Health, SVS 2011) for mortality by diarrhea and World Health Organization health statistics (WHO 2010) for child mortality.

mortality have improved more than twice as much as in the average country in Latin America and the Caribbean (table 3.1). Among select countries of similar income level,[17] only Peru and Turkey increased life expectancy and reduced infant mortality more (around 16.5 percent for life expectancy and 76 percent for infant mortality).

However, other indicators paint a less positive picture. For maternal mortality, official figures indicate a high and stagnant rate in the last 20 years, around 50 deaths per 100,000 live births, in a country where more than 90 percent of births

Table 3.1 Change in Health Outcomes in Brazil and Comparable Countries, 1985–2009
percentage change

Country or group of countries	Life expectancy	Infant mortality
Brazil	15.5	−71.3
Latin America and the Caribbean	7.1	−33.2
Middle-income countries	6.1	−28.5
China and India	11.1	−60.5
Best performers in group[a]	16.5	−76.3

Sources: IBGE 2004; Ministry of Health data (Ministry of Health, SVS 2011); World Bank 2011.
a. Best performers are Peru and Turkey.

Figure 3.21 Maternal Mortality in Brazil and Latin America and the Caribbean, 1990–2009

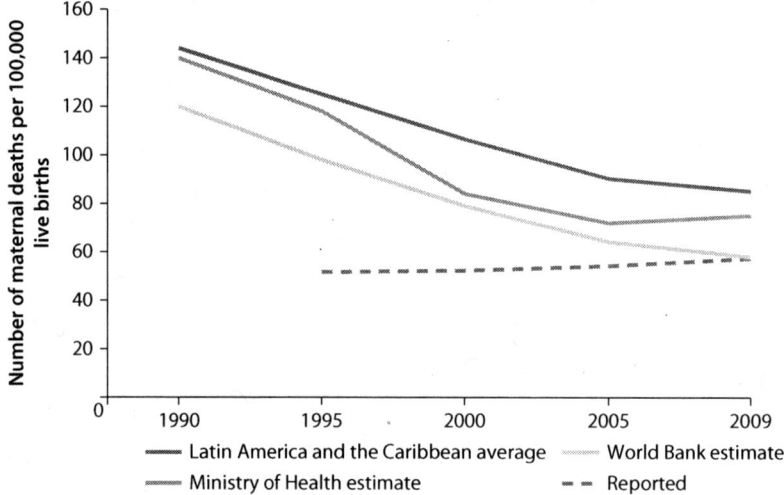

Sources: Ministry of Health, SVS 2011 and previous years; World Bank 2011.

take place in a hospital setting. In comparison with other countries, Brazil's adjusted rate runs below the regional average, but is twice as high or more as in Chile and Turkey (26), Malaysia (31), or China and the Russian Federation (38–39).[18] Brazil is unlikely to meet the Millennium Development Goal for maternal mortality (35 deaths per 100,000 live births). However, focused studies suggest that the apparent stagnation of the maternal mortality rate may be the result of improvements in the identification and recording of maternal deaths.[19] Adjusted estimates based on regression techniques, by both the Ministry of Health and the World Bank, show significant reductions in maternal deaths over the last 20 years, from 140 to 75 deaths per 100,000 live births (figure 3.21).[20] However, even based on these estimates, the maternal mortality rate remains relatively high.

Some preventable causes of mortality or morbidity are on the rise. Dengue and malaria, for instance, fluctuate widely year-to-year without showing signs of being under effective control. Mortality from traffic accidents declined between 1996 and 2000, but has remained stable or increased since then, at around

18.5 deaths per 1 million population (Ministry of Health 2010b). Mortality from homicides doubled, from 14 deaths per 100,000 population in 1980 to 28 in 2006 and has decreased slightly since then.

Inequalities in Health Outcomes

Life expectancy, infant mortality, and other outcomes improved substantially in all states, but at quite different speeds. Geographic inequalities in health outcomes were significantly reduced, with northeastern states benefiting the most (Bahia, Ceará, Pernambuco, Piauí, and Rio Grande do Norte). These states had the lowest baseline values. Gains in life expectancy varied from 6.2 years in Pernambuco to 3.3 in Amapá, with an average of 4.6 (figure 3.22). The mean deviation in life expectancy decreased from 2.35 years to 1.90. The same is true of infant mortality, although the best-performing states are not exactly the same.

The reduction in mean deviation was even greater: from 14.49 to 6.05 deaths per 1,000 live births. The poorer northeastern and northern regions experienced the largest reductions, although they continue to have higher rates (figure 3.23). The achievement of nearly full child immunization coverage in all regions, improvements in child nutrition (which were more pronounced in the Northeast), and implementation and coverage of the ESF and other programs that prioritized poor regions and population groups contributed to this trend, as mentioned elsewhere in this report.

Figure 3.24 further illustrates these trends, this time across regions. The difference between the regions with the highest and the lowest infant mortality rates—Northeast and South—dropped from 3:1 to 2:1 during the period.

Disparities in health outcomes have been reduced not only geographically, but also across socioeconomic groups. For instance, figure 3.25 shows that the reduction in the infant mortality rate was much greater among low-income groups, contributing to the convergence of different income groups to around 20 deaths out of 1,000 live births by the mid-2000s.

Has the SUS Contributed to Improved Health Outcomes?

While the improved outcomes and lower inequalities in health are good news, these gains are attributable at least in part to developments outside the health system: access to safe water and sanitation, quality food and education, and the economic situation of households.[21] Nearly a quarter of the population is covered by private insurance and another 15 percent do not use the SUS as their regular source of care, which complicates the picture further. Finally, several broad public health programs that are linked only partially to the SUS reforms have also contributed to improvements. These include, for example, a Ministry of Health program promoting breast-feeding, which was initiated in 1981. As a result of this program, the mean duration of breast-feeding increased from 2.5 months in the mid-1970s to 14 months in 2006–07 (Victora *et al.* 2011).

Have the SUS reforms contributed to improving health outcomes? This is very difficult to answer with certainty because reforms were implemented

Figure 3.22 Life Expectancy and Infant Mortality in Brazil, by State, 1994 (or 1995) and 2007 (or 2009)

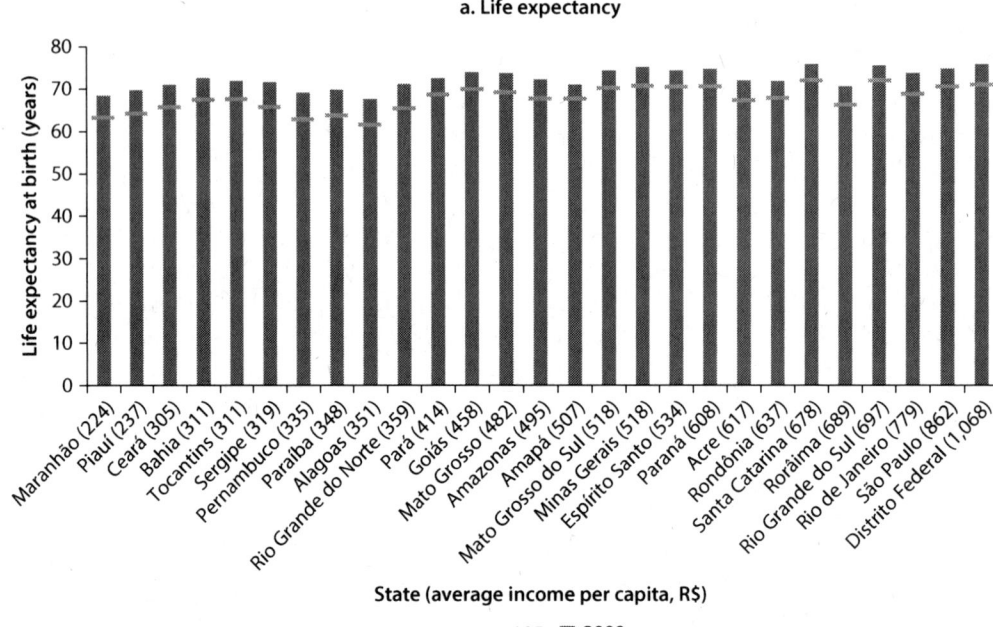

a. Life expectancy

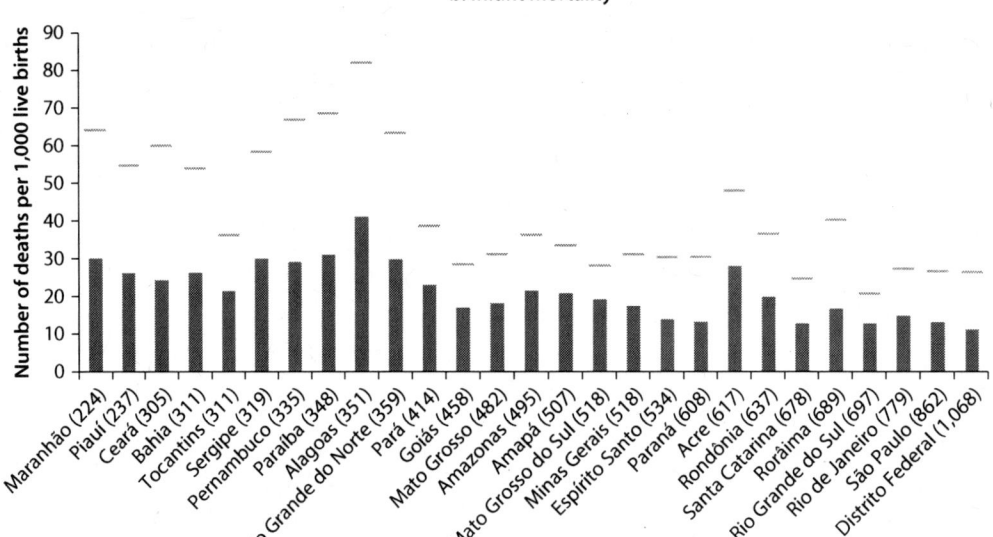

b. Infant mortality

Source: Couttolenc 2011, based on Ministry of Health data.

Figure 3.23 Link between Health Outcomes and Average Income per Capita in Brazil, 1994 (or 1995) and 2007 (or 2009)

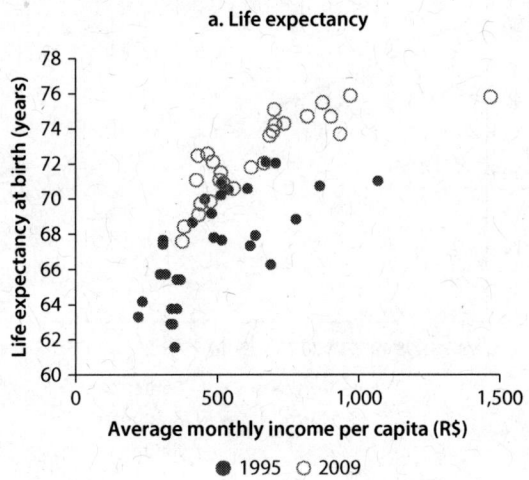

a. Life expectancy

● 1995 ○ 2009

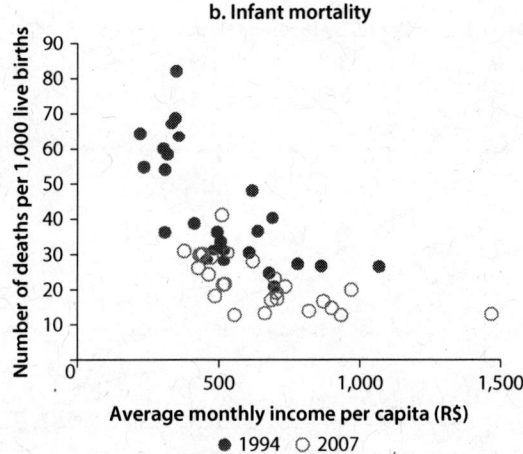

b. Infant mortality

● 1994 ○ 2007

Sources: Ministry of Health, DATASUS data for life expectancy and infant mortality; IPEAData from IBGE for state income.

nationwide and the quality and consistency of administrative data from the program are problematic. There is, however, some convincing evidence from studies of avoidable mortality and evaluations of the ESF that the SUS has played an important role in improving health outcomes.

Avoidable Mortality

One way to identify the contribution of the health system in improving health outcomes is to look at trends in avoidable (or amenable) mortality—that is, deaths that could have been avoided in the presence of timely and effective

Figure 3.24 Infant Mortality in Brazil, by Region, 1997–2007

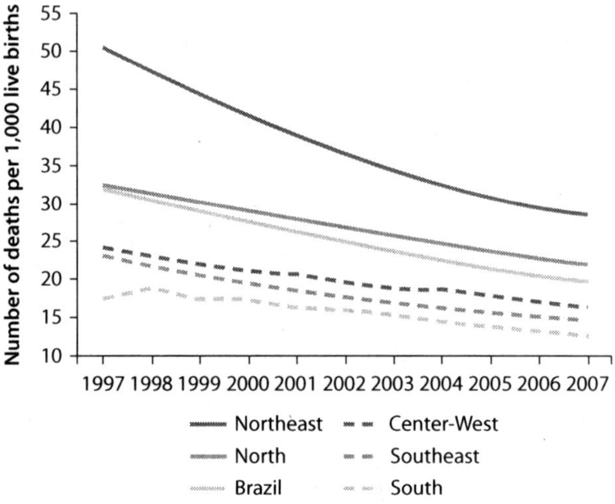

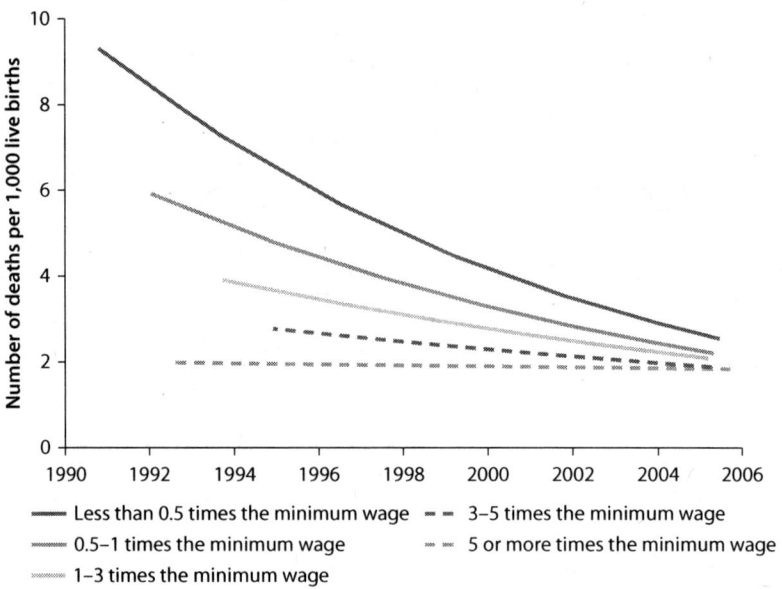

Source: Rocha 2011, based on Ministry of Health data.

Figure 3.25 Infant Mortality in Brazil, by Income Group, 1990–2006

Source: IBGE, PNAD for various years.

health care. This approach is based on data from national death registers, which record the cause of death based on standardized classifications of disease.[22] Mortality from specific conditions is then defined as avoidable, and this permits an analysis of trends and patterns (for example, variation between countries or regions) of mortality that could have been avoided. The premise of this analysis is that improvements or spatial differences in the coverage or effectiveness of the health system over time will be reflected in the data on avoidable mortality.[23]

Various studies of avoidable mortality in Brazil suggest that the SUS has played an important role in improving outcomes. For instance, Malta *et al.* (2010) examined trends in avoidable mortality in infants (children under one year of age) during the period of 1997–2006. They found a significant decline in both avoidable deaths (37 percent) and deaths from ill-defined causes (75 percent), indicating improved access to health care, but stable mortality from other causes (a reduction of 2.2 percent). This is likely to be driven at least in part by improvements in coverage and quality of the health system. For instance, mortality from pneumonia fell 52.7 percent, with effective primary care likely to have played an important role. However, other factors, particularly improvements in living conditions and public health interventions that affect the incidence of different health conditions, are also likely to have played a role. While the study presents a positive picture of the health system overall, it also reports an *increase* of 28 percent in mortality avoidable through adequate prenatal care. This is hard to reconcile with improvements in coverage of prenatal care, but the authors speculate that poor quality of prenatal care may have played a role.[24]

Along similar lines, Abreu, Cesar, and Franca (2007) studied trends in avoidable mortality for children and adults between 1983 and 2002, using data from 117 municipalities. Comparing the periods 1983–92 and 1993–2002, they found that avoidable mortality declined significantly, while mortality from other causes remained stable. They also noted a significant difference between women and men, with ischemic heart disease accounting for most of this difference (there is also a large gender difference in mortality from other causes, most likely the result of different rates of death due to violence and accidents; see also Abreu, Cesar, and Franca 2009).

The studies of avoidable mortality in Brazil are unfortunately not comparable with the studies from OECD countries, so international comparisons are not possible at this point. However, the significant decline in avoidable mortality over the last couple of decades indicates that the geographic expansion of the health system and the increased focus on primary care are contributing to improved health outcomes, although other factors may also be playing a role.

Impact of the ESF on Health Outcomes

Evaluations of the ESF provide another piece of the puzzle. An early evaluation of the ESF (Ministry of Health 2000), which surveyed the 1,219 municipalities that had implemented the program as of 1998, found that the ESF was associated with a dramatic increase in health promotion and prevention activities, including prenatal care, family planning, cancer screening, and chronic disease management.[25] However, simple comparisons between municipalities with and without ESF are problematic, as the rollout and expansion of the program have, to some extent, been systematically related to local conditions (health needs, economic development, political circumstances, and so forth). Moreover, the impact of the program is likely to depend on how long it has been implemented and the level of coverage achieved.

World Bank (2002) made an early attempt to deal with these issues in evaluating the impact of the ESF. The study compared changes in outcomes between 1995 and 1998 for municipalities with and without the ESF, finding some evidence that the ESF was reducing infant mortality rates and hospital admissions.

More recent studies have been able to achieve larger samples and use longer time periods to study the program. For instance, Macinko et al. (2006) found that implementation of the ESF was associated with significant reductions in infant mortality, diarrhea incidence among children, hospitalization for strokes, and acute respiratory infections in the period between 1990 and 2002. For example, a 10 percent increase in ESF coverage was associated with a 4.5 percent decrease ($p < 0.01$) in the infant mortality rate. Along similar lines, Aquino, Oliveira, and Barreto (2009), using data from 1996 to 2004, found reductions in the infant mortality rate ranging from 13 to 22 percent depending on the level of coverage (coverage of less than 30, 30–69.9, or 70 percent or more).

Rocha and Soares (2009) used both administrative and survey data to study the impact of the ESF on health outcomes (mortality) and household behaviors (schooling, fertility, and labor supply). They also found a significant impact on health, with eight years of implementation being associated with a 20 percent reduction in infant mortality. They reported notable heterogeneity in impact, with large and significant reductions in infant mortality in the North and Northeast and no significant impacts in other parts of the country.[26]

Given how the ESF has been implemented, it is impossible to determine the impact of the program with certainty. Nonetheless, taken together, these studies provide a strong indication that the rollout of the ESF has contributed to a reduction in mortality, in particular among children and in the North and Northeast.

Out-of-Pocket Payments and Financial Protection

The principle of universality is related not only to the use of services, but also to the extent that individuals are able to access services without financial distress. Hence, effective financial protection is considered an important goal and one of the criteria against which the performance of a health system is typically measured.

Progress with regard to financial protection is typically assessed using data on household health spending over a defined period (for example, one month) based on household surveys that record expenditures on both private health insurance and direct out-of-pocket payments for drugs, health services from private providers, or copayments in public facilities (in cases where such co-payments are levied).

As noted in chapter 2, private spending still accounts for a significant share of overall health spending. While the share of private spending on health is an important variable, it is not necessarily the best guide for assessing the burden that households face in paying for health care. For this, detailed analysis of

Figure 3.26 Share of the Household Budget Spent on Health in Brazil, 1987–2003

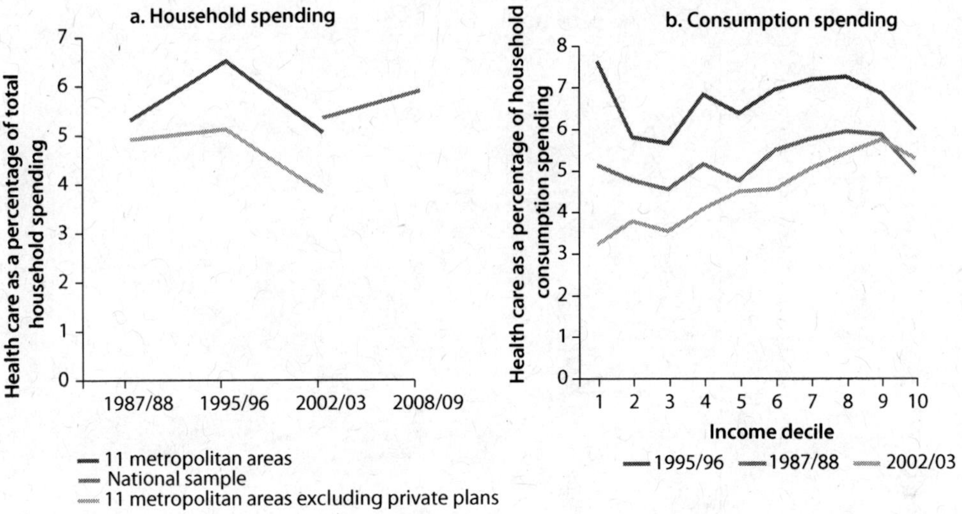

a. Household spending

Health care as a percentage of total household spending

(y-axis: 0–7)

x-axis: 1987/88   1995/96   2002/03   2008/09

— 11 metropolitan areas
— National sample
⋯ 11 metropolitan areas excluding private plans

b. Consumption spending

Health care as a percentage of household consumption spending

(y-axis: 0–8)

Income decile: 1 2 3 4 5 6 7 8 9 10

— 1995/96   — 1987/88   ⋯ 2002/03

Sources: Estimates from 11 metropolitan areas and disaggregations by decile are from Diniz *et al.* 2007; National estimates are from POF survey reports (IBGE 2002, 2010).

household survey data provide a more meaningful perspective, as it allows an assessment of how health expenditures relate to income and how they are distributed across households.

Available household survey data (*Pesquisa dos Orçamentos Familiares*, POF), which offer data points ranging from 1987 to 2008, suggest that there has been little change over time in the share of total household spending dedicated to health, with estimates ranging from 5 to 7 percent (figure 3.26). There was a notable increase in the burden of spending between 1987 and 1995, but this trend was reversed between 1995 and 2002. While the share of total household spending dedicated to health was similar across the income distribution in 1987–88 and 1995–96, the share of household spending on health at the lower end of the income distribution declined notably in 2002–03.

While household spending on health remained stable as a share of the household budget over the last 20 years, the composition of spending changed dramatically (figure 3.27). Charges for services (consultations, hospitalization, and dental care) accounted for more than half of spending in 1987–88, but this share declined to 20 percent in 2008–09. Over the same period, spending on private plans (in particular between 1987 and 1995) and on drugs rose. Indeed, the rise in spending on private plans accounts for most of the rise in the share of the household budget spent on health in the early 1990s, with drugs playing an important role in the late 1990s and 2000s.

Of course, the composition of household spending on health and its change over time vary significantly across socioeconomic groups. For the bottom deciles of the income distribution, spending on drugs accounts for between 60 and

Figure 3.27 Composition of Household Spending on Health in Brazil, 1987–2009

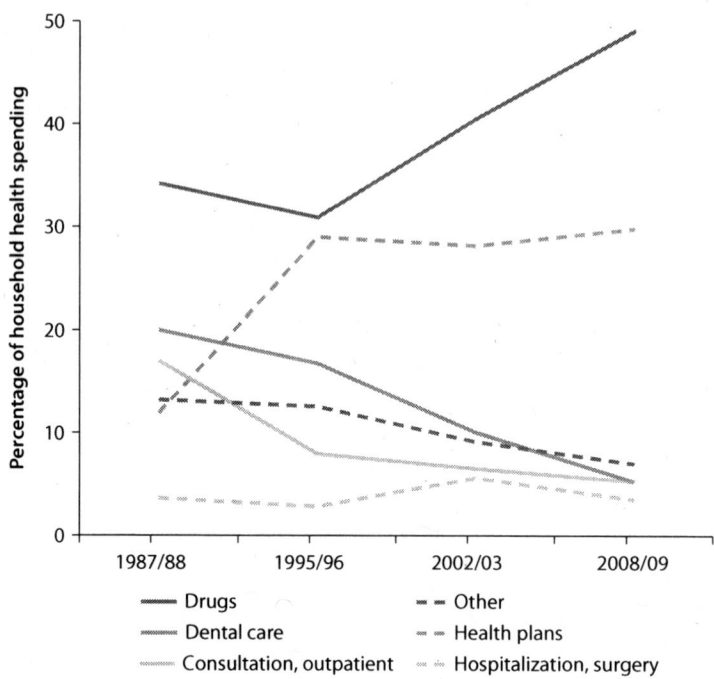

Sources: All estimates are from the Pesquisa dos Orçamentos Familiares (POF). Data for 1987–88 and 1995–96 are from Medici 2003; data for subsequent years are from POF survey reports (IBGE 2002, 2010).

70 percent of total health spending, while spending on private health plans accounts for only 5–10 percent. Conversely, at the upper end of the income distribution, 35–45 percent of total health spending is on private health plans, while only 25–35 percent is on drugs (figure 3.28). While the share of health spending on private plans has a strong income gradient, it increased notably across the income distribution between 1987 and 1995.

The average share of health spending in total consumption provides an important perspective on the burden of health expenditures for households, in particular, on whether a large share of it is in the form of out-of-pocket spending. However, the distribution of spending across households also matters, in particular, the extent to which some households spend a very large share of their income on health (referred to as "catastrophic health expenditures").[27] Because estimates of catastrophic spending depend critically on methodological choices (how income or disposable income is defined and the cutoff for catastrophic spending that is applied) and on the data at hand (in particular the comprehensiveness of income and health spending measures), there is a wide range of estimates for Brazil.

Perhaps the most systematic effort to assess the incidence of catastrophic health is a study by Diniz *et al.* (2007), based on data from the POF.[28] Using a cutoff of 40 percent and total income minus food expenditures as a measure of disposable income, they found an incidence of catastrophic spending of

Figure 3.28 Household Spending on Drugs and Private Health Plans in Brazil, by Income Distribution, 1987–2003

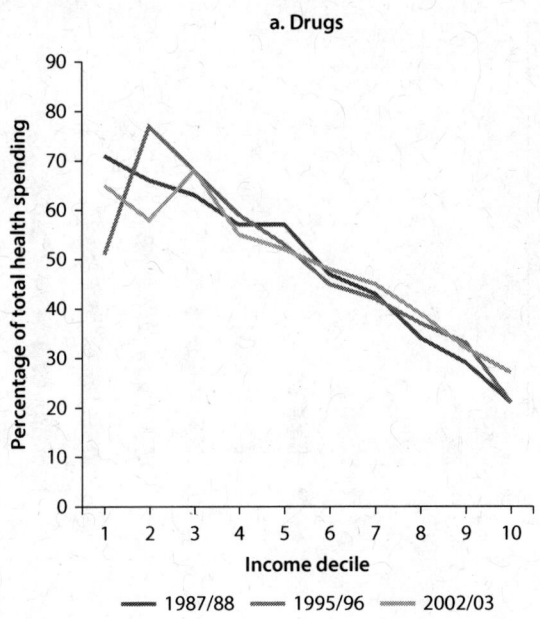

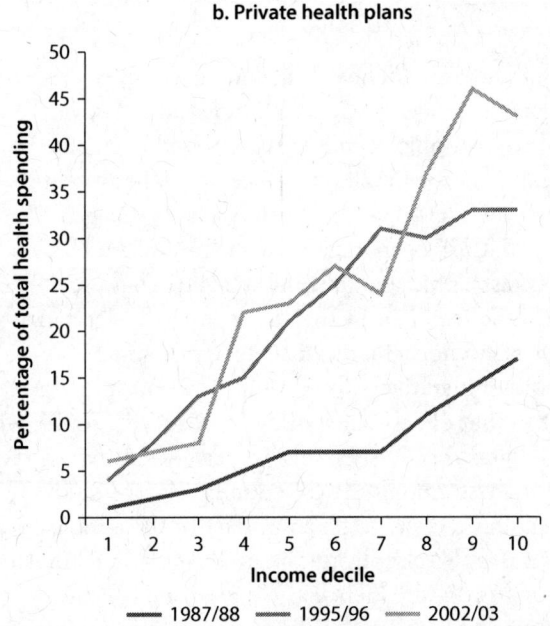

Sources: Diniz *et al.* 2007, based on the Pesquisa dos Orçamentos Familiares (POF) (using a consistent subsample from 11 metropolitan areas).

Figure 3.29 Incidence of Catastrophic Spending on Health in Select Latin American Countries, Various Years, 2002–08

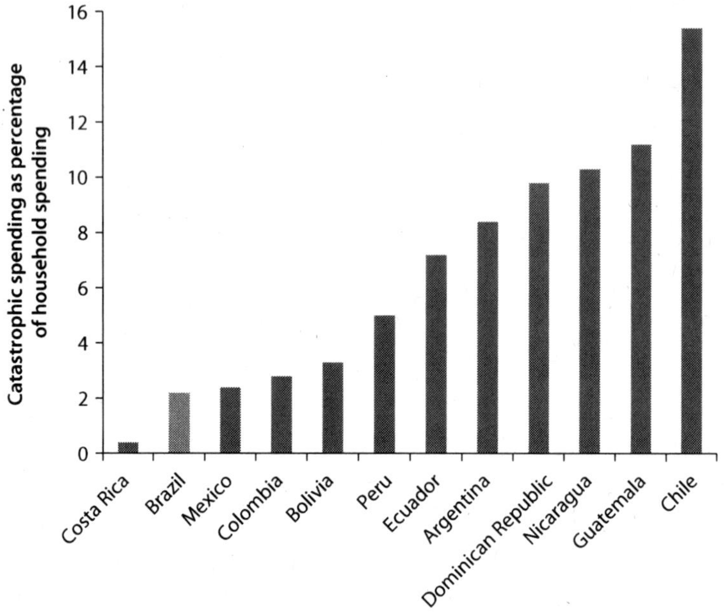

Source: Data from Knaul et al. 2011.
Note: Data for Brazil are for 2002–03. Data for other countries are for various years ranging from 2002 to 2008.

2.2 percent if all household health spending is considered and 1.9 percent if spending on private plans is excluded. No studies provide evidence on how the incidence of catastrophic spending has evolved over time.

Using the same data for Brazil, but a slightly different approach, Knaul et al. (2011) compared the incidence of catastrophic spending in 12 countries in the Latin America and Caribbean region. They found that Brazil has one of the lowest levels of catastrophic spending in the region (figure 3.29). Similar to many other countries in the region, catastrophic spending is significantly higher among poorer households and households with elderly members.

The finding of comparatively low levels of catastrophic spending in Brazil is in stark contrast to that of an earlier study by Xu et al. (2003), which found that the incidence of catastrophic spending in Brazil—estimated at 10.3 percent— was the second highest among the 59 countries in the study. This high level of catastrophic spending is likely to be an artifact of the data used, and subsequent studies have been unable to replicate the findings using nationally representative data (see Diniz et al. 2007).[29] Hence, there are good reasons to believe that catastrophic health spending in Brazil is low both in absolute terms and relative to that of other countries in the region.[30]

Overall, there is no clear evidence that the share of health in total household spending has been declining over time. The incidence of catastrophic spending appears to be relatively low in Brazil, but health spending undoubtedly continues to be a significant burden for many Brazilian households. A large share of this burden is due to spending on private health plans and drugs.

In the case of private health plans, these expenditures are voluntary and comprise a prepayment of health expenditures incurred at a later date. However, households with insurance plans do not necessarily have a lower incidence of catastrophic health spending; if anything, the opposite is true (Barros, Bastos, and Damaso 2011; Bos and Waters 2008; Knaul et al. 2011). The primary function of private plans seems to be to ensure timely access to health services and perhaps higher quality. High demand for private plans indicates that the SUS is failing to deliver on some of its promises and raises important equity concerns. Private plans may also suffer from moral hazard on both the demand and supply sides, such that not all services provided are appropriate and necessary. Insofar as this is the case, high levels of private spending on health plans raise efficiency concerns.

The government has taken many measures to reduce household spending on drugs, introducing the National Medicines Policy in 1998, gradually expanding the Popular Pharmacies Program since 2004, and steadily increasing government spending on pharmaceuticals (Vieira 2009). These strategies appear to be working. In real terms, household spending on drugs declined between 1995 and 2002, from R$73 to R$53, and then increased slightly to R$59 in 2008 (Garcia et al. 2011).[31] Moreover, at least in areas where the population has good access to the SUS, the SUS provides a large share of the drugs consumed. For instance, in a study of households covered by the ESF in Porto Alegre, Rio Grande Sul, the SUS provided for free nearly 70 percent of all the medicine consumed (80 percent for the bottom quintile; 31 percent for the top two quintiles; Bertoldi et al. 2011).

Nonetheless, high levels of household spending on drugs persist for a range of reasons. First, availability of drugs in public pharmacies remains a problem (Bertoldi et al. 2012), and studies have found that sometimes as high as 40 percent of the drugs prescribed in public primary care were not available when needed (Naves and Silver 2005; Santos and Nitrini 2004). Evidence from the Pesquisa Nacional por Amostra de Domicílios (PNAD) also suggests that, although the supply of free drugs in the SUS has increased over time, in 2008, more than half of the drugs prescribed by SUS providers were not received for free (figure 3.30). Second, much of drug expenditures appear to be for drugs that are not on the SUS list of essential drugs, typically prescribed by non-SUS providers or self-medicated (Bertoldi et al. 2009, 2011; figure 3.31). This raises important questions about whether the rationing of drugs in the SUS is rational and whether drugs not on the list have demonstrated health benefits. Finally, drug prices for key drugs appear to be comparatively high in Brazil (Bertoldi et al. 2012).

Public Perceptions of and Satisfaction with the Health System

The primary goals of the health system are to improve health outcomes and provide financial protection. However, most people (and policy makers) also consider satisfaction and responsiveness important intrinsic objectives. Although

Figure 3.30 Access to Dental Care and Medications from the SUS in Brazil, 1981–2008

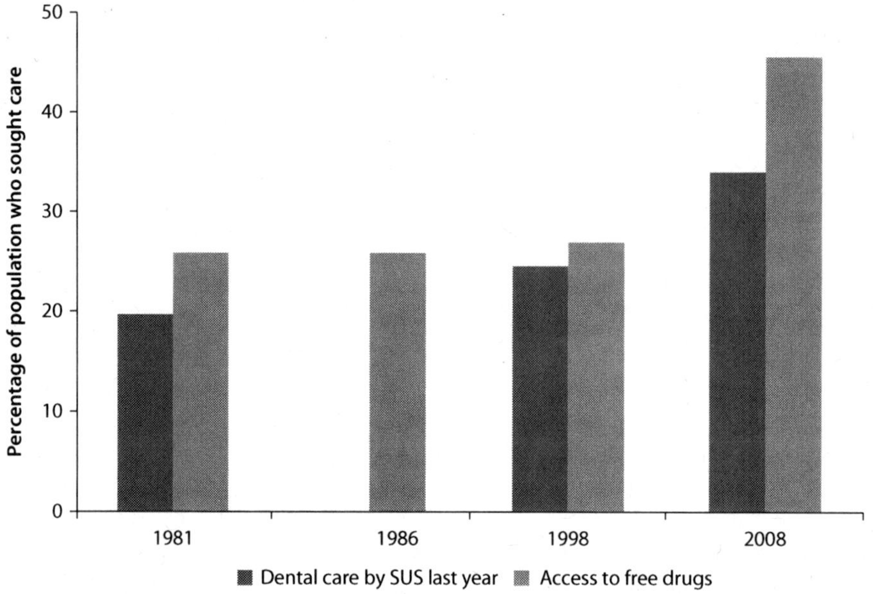

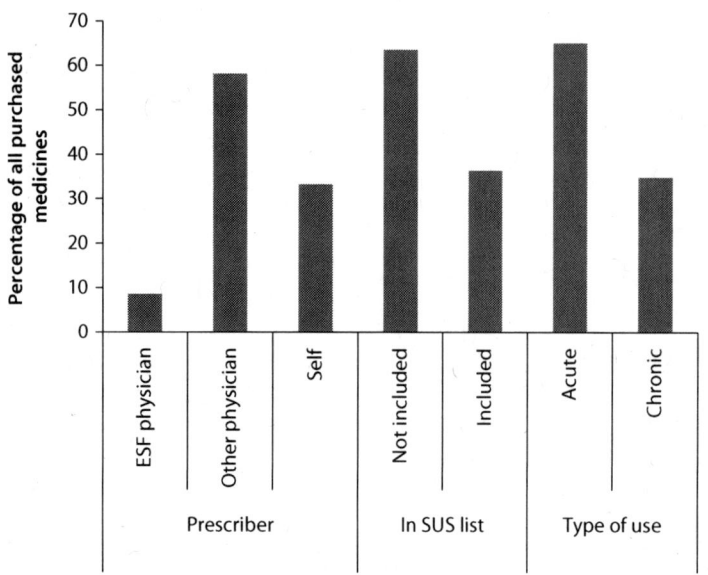

Source: IBGE, PNAD for 1981–2008.
Note: SUS = Sistema Único de Saúde. Access to dental care is defined as the proportion of individuals seeking dental care during the previous year who were treated by an SUS dental facility or professional; access to free drugs is defined as the proportion of SUS users prescribed medications during their last consultation who received their medications free either fully or in part.

Figure 3.31 Drugs Paid for Out-of-Pocket in Brazil, by SUS List, Type of Prescriber, and Use, 2008

Source: Data from Bertoldi et al. 2009.
Note: ESF = Family Health Strategy, SUS = Sistema Único de Saúde. Percentage of all purchased medicines (which account for 41 percent of all medicines consumed), based on a sample of 2,988 individuals in Porto Alegre (30-day recall).

important, satisfaction and responsiveness are difficult to measure in systematic and consistent ways.

This section does not aim to provide a comprehensive review of the literature on satisfaction with the health system in Brazil. However, recent opinion polls provide an important perspective on current health system challenges. For instance, a study by the National Confederation of Industry (Confederação Nacional da Indústria, CNI) reports that 61 percent of the population consider public health services to be bad or terrible, with 85 percent seeing no change or a worsening over the last three years (CNI 2012).[32] The problems that are most commonly reported are delay in access or treatment and lack of doctors. The main strike against public hospitals, which were rated worse than private hospitals, is waiting times for consultations and for exams.

A recent survey by Datafolha reached similar conclusions (Folha de São Paulo 2012). According to the study, a growing share of the population considers health to be the "main problem in the country" (39 percent), up from 28 percent in 2010 and significantly higher than in the early 2000s.[33]

In contrast, a study by the Institute of Applied Economic Research (Instituto de Pesquisa Econômica Aplicada, IPEA) (IPEA 2011) provides a more positive assessment, with only 28.5 percent of users thinking that SUS services are bad or very bad (28.9 percent found them good or very good). The study found some variation across different parts of the SUS, with the ESF receiving the most positive assessment and basic care units and emergency care being considered the worst. In terms of key problems, the survey responses resonate with the findings of other studies, highlighting the lack of doctors and long waiting times for hospital or referral services as key concerns. However, the survey also found that many individuals consider having a private health plan as very important, with getting more rapid access to services being the most important reason. A similar finding was reported in a study that sampled 1,626 individuals with health plans and 1,627 individuals without plans (IESS 2011). Nearly all sampled individuals without health plans (88 percent) considered having a plan as "important" or "very important." When asked to rank health plans among 12 other assets, goods, or services, health plans were ranked second, ahead of a car, life insurance, new household appliances, and a computer, with "own house" being the only item ranked as more important.

Opinion polls are often based on relatively small samples, and answers tend to be very sensitive to how questions are asked. Results should therefore be treated with some care. Moreover, some surveys are not able to distinguish dissatisfaction with the SUS from satisfaction with the broader health system, including private health plans and providers. Nonetheless, the findings from several polls reveal a high level of dissatisfaction with the SUS and highlight problems related to access and long waiting times as key issues, factors that contribute to the continued (perhaps growing) demand for private health insurance.[34] These results have to be contrasted with more positive assessments in other surveys.

Of course, given the nearly limitless demand for health care, all countries struggle to meet expectations. Yet dissatisfaction with the health system is

Figure 3.32 Satisfaction with the Health System in Select Countries, by GDP per Capita, 2010

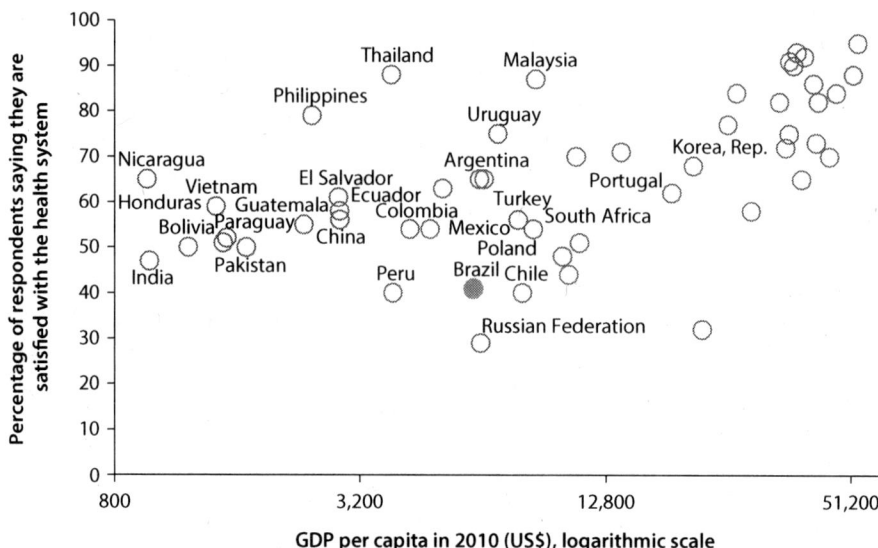

Sources: Data on satisfaction with the health system from the Gallup World Poll; data on GDP from World Bank 2010.
Note: GDP = gross domestic product.

particularly high in Brazil.[35] In a recently conducted round of the Gallup World
Poll, which asked randomly selected households across a wide range of countries
about their satisfaction with public services and other issues, only 40 percent of
Brazilians were satisfied with the health system. This is significantly lower than
in many other middle-income countries that have achieved or made significant
strides toward universal coverage in recent years (for example, Malaysia,
Thailand, Turkey, or Uruguay; figure 3.32).

Notes

1. Through the 1970s and 1980s, INAMPS gradually expanded its coverage from the
   initial target group of workers employed in the urban formal sector by including rural
   workers (1969–71) and then domestic and self-employed workers (1972–73) and by
   dropping the requirement to present a Social Security card to be treated in its
   network.

2. There are large variations in the data regarding coverage over the years. For example,
   data on private health insurance fluctuated when the regulatory agency (Agência
   Nacional de Saúde Suplementar, ANS) was established and began collecting sector
   data in 2000; the ANS does not collect data on self-managed plans offered directly by
   employers through their human resource or other department. These types of plans
   largely cover civil servants, who account for some 10 million workers and dependents.
   Another discontinuity in the data appears in the proportion of out-of-pocket expenditures between 1981 and 1986 (20 and 34 percent, respectively).

3. The figures for medical consultation and basic care are not exactly comparable over
   time due to changes in classification in SUS information systems; however, these
   changes do not affect significantly the general trends observed. The high and rising

number of primary health care procedures per capita reflects not only the increase in coverage and supply, but also the increasing detail in recording and counting the different types of services provided. More than 1,000 procedures are recorded and counted, including medical and other professional consultations, home visits and outreach activities, treatments and therapies, drug administration, immunizations, diagnostic tests, and others. The list was substantially changed in 1999, which makes comparisons over time imprecise.

4. OECD health data for 2011 and Word Bank, World Development Indicators for various years.

5. IBGE's annual household survey (*Pesquisa Nacional por Amostra de Domicílios*, PNAD) is the main source of data on this issue, but they suffer from some inconsistency in the definition of variables over the years. Specifically, computing and comparing the proportion of people seeking (or not seeking) care when ill is not possible since the PNAD of 1986 defined sickness as "having a health problem in the last two weeks," while the surveys since 1998 defined it as "having to interrupt daily activities due to a health problem." To address this problem, we computed the proportion of people who did not seek care when they felt they needed it, excluding those who did not seek care because they felt they did not need it; although this approach is not rigorous or precise, it provides the best approach to estimating general difficulties related to access. For a detailed discussion, see Osorio, Servo, and Piola (2011).

6. The relative importance of these reasons varies widely across states. For instance, distance and transportation are important in the low-density states of the northern region, while economic reasons are more important in poorer states (but this is where they decreased most in importance). Reasons related to facility characteristics were consistently more important in the richer states of the Southeast, South, and Center-West.

7. Late diagnosis (stages three and four) was even more common for certain forms of cancer, such as lung cancer.

8. Hospital registry data present a slightly different picture, with a median waiting time of 70.3 days and 38.4 percent of patients waiting less than 30 days. The registries are intended to be national in scope, but currently only cover certain states and selected hospitals. More than 80 percent of the data come from Minas Gerais, Paraná, Rio de Janeiro, Rio Grande do Sul, and Santa Catarina. There are also serious data quality issues.

9. Based on norms established in Portaria SAS/MS 741/2005, indicating the expected number of cancer patients requiring surgery, chemotherapy, and radiation therapy, the report finds a deficit in treatment capacity, with significant geographic differences. The volume of services is also lower than needed as defined by the norms, with the SUS only supplying 66 percent of needed radiation therapy procedures and 34.5 percent of needed cancer surgeries.

10. At one level, this is likely to be an overestimate, as some patients may have been waiting for a shorter period. However, the data do not include patients who were unable to secure a referral or who gave up trying to access specialist care.

11. The concept of "effective coverage" has been coined to capture both the access and quality dimensions, referring to the extent to which potential health gains are realized.

12. Quality assurance programs are numerous in Brazil. For instance, several major hospital accreditation systems are in place: the National Accreditation Organization

(Organização Nacional de Acreditação); the hospital quality assurance initiative sponsored by the Medical Association of São Paulo (Controle da Qualidade Hospitalar); the Brazilian accreditation initiative (Consórcio Brasileiro de Acreditação) supported by the U.S. Joint Commission on Accreditation of Healthcare Organizations; and the National Quality Award (Premio Nacional da Qualidade), a multisector quality assurance initiative of the National Quality Foundation. In addition, the country has among the largest number of hospitals in the United Nations Children's Fund's Baby Friendly Hospital Initiative. However, quality assurance efforts tend to be unsystematic and fragmented, and there have been few evaluations of their effectiveness to date. Currently, less than 5 percent of existing hospitals are accredited by any of these systems. Such low buy-in appears to be related to the absence of strong incentives for hospitals to engage in systematic quality improvement and accreditation and to the absence of systematic and coherent national policies on the issue.

13. In 1980, INAMPS reduced the amount reimbursed for a Cesarean section, which used to be higher than for normal deliveries; the SUS established a ceiling of 40 percent in the proportion of Cesarean sections in 1998 and then reduced it to 30 percent in 2000 (Victora *et al.* 2011).

14. There are, of course, broader allocative issues—for example, concerning the balance between prevention (including activities outside the health sector) and curative services. This issue is difficult to tackle at the health system level, but can usefully be addressed in relation to specific conditions or health risks. It is not addressed in this report given the limited evidence that is available.

15. For Brazil, Couttolenc, Dias, and Nicolella (2004); La Forgia and Couttolenc (2008); and SES-MG (2005). For Spain, Caminal, Starfield, and Sanchez (2004). For the United States, Vali (2001) and Axene and McQuillian (1999).

16. Using data from the World Bank (2010) changes the numbers a bit (an increase of 12.8 percent), but not the trend.

17. The reference countries include five from Latin America (Argentina, Chile, Colombia, Mexico, and Peru), the other emerging BRICS (Russia, India, China, and South Africa), and two Asian countries (Malaysia and Thailand).

18. WHO, Healthstats estimates.

19. In recent years, technical committees for the review of deaths of women in reproductive years have been established in all states, covering 40 percent of all deaths in 2009; this effort is likely to improve reporting.

20. World Bank estimates offer rates of 120 deaths per 100,000 live births in 1985 and 58 in 2009, a decline of 51.7 percent.

21. For instance, access to safe water increased steadily from 57.8 percent of the population in 1981 to 91.5 percent in 2007, while access to sanitation increased from 37.6 to 71.6 percent during the period. Economic conditions also improved substantially in spite of several economic crises, with mean household income per capita increasing 50.9 percent in real terms from 1981 to 2009 (from R$467,75 to R$705,72). Perhaps more important, the proportion of individuals living in poverty (that is, with less than one minimum wage salary per month) nearly halved.

22. The list of conditions for which mortality is considered amenable has varied significantly over time and across studies. In part, this reflects the introduction of new technology, but also the extent to which studies have focused on personal health care services alone or have also taken into account broader primary prevention interventions. For details, see Nolte and McKee (2003).

23. Of course, changes in avoidable mortality reflect both changes in incidence and effectiveness of health care (treatment as well as secondary and tertiary prevention). Some care is needed in interpreting the data. Nolte and McKee (2003) note, "Avoidable mortality was never intended to be more than an indicator of potential weaknesses in health care that can then be investigated in more depth."

24. Two recent studies focusing on a cohort of children in Pelotas (Gorgot et al. 2011; Santos et al. 2011) found that most of the mortality in children was avoidable, largely through adequate maternal care during pregnancy (70 percent of deaths), and that most deaths occurred in the first year of life (92 percent). The increase in premature deaths and poor prenatal care were contributing factors. They also documented a socioeconomic gradient, with children born to women in the lowest quintile having a three times higher probability of dying from avoidable causes than those born to women in the highest quintile, in part because preterm births are nearly twice as high in the lowest quintile. Effective cessation of smoking and provision of progesterone to high-risk women could help to reduce mortality. The increase in mortality that could be avoided through effective prenatal care may also be partly due to an increase in maternal conditions that affect the fetus (for example, diabetes) and improved diagnosis and more accurate classification of deaths.

25. Similar findings were reported in Ministry of Health (2008).

26. For the Northeast (and, to a lesser extent, the North), they also found a significant impact on mortality for other age groups. Moreover, the program was associated with significant increases in schooling and labor market participation.

27. There are various approaches to measuring the incidence of catastrophic spending (O'Donnell et al. 2008). Xu et al. (2003) considers health spending to be catastrophic if it accounts for more than 40 percent of disposable income, with disposable income defined as total consumption minus spending on food (or an estimated "subsistence" amount for households with low food spending). Other studies use total income or consumption as a denominator, but apply a different cutoff point (typically between 5 and 20 percent). While most studies consider only direct out-of-pocket spending in estimates of catastrophic spending, some include spending on health plans on the grounds that these expenditures contribute to the overall burden of health spending (for example, Bos and Waters 2008).

28. Diniz et al. (2007) is based on data for 1987–88, 1995–96, and 2002–03, but the authors only estimate the incidence of catastrophic spending for 2002–03. The sample design changed significantly between rounds. The 1987–88 and 1995–96 rounds sampled the population in 11 metropolitan areas that account for approximately 30 percent of the Brazilian population; the 2002–03 sample is nationally representative. There were also differences in the timing (and reference periods) of the different surveys. Finally, the 2002–03 survey questionnaires included a more detailed aggregation of health spending and also captured nonmonetary spending. In order to ensure that the data from the respective rounds were comparable, the authors worked with a subsample of the 2002–03 survey, transformed all amounts into real values, and mapped the spending categories in the 2002–03 survey and those used in earlier rounds.

29. The estimates of Xu et al. (2003) are based on the 1996–97 Living Standards Survey, which surveyed around 5,000 households in 10 geographic areas. The sample is considerably smaller than for the POF, and the survey is not nationally representative. Furthermore, the measures of total consumption (denominator) only include expenditures; they do not capture imputed rent, home production, and other in-kind

elements of consumption. Using the methodology of Xu *et al.* (2003), but with total consumption and a 40 percent cutoff, Diniz *et al.* (2007) found that only 0.6 percent of households have catastrophic spending. Using monetary income as a proxy for expenditure—the closest they can get to the denominator used by Xu *et al.* (2003), catastrophic spending is estimated at 6 percent.

30. Other studies using the same data have reached different conclusions. These differences are largely due to the way in which income (and disposable income) is measured. For instance, Campino (2011) found that 7 percent of households in the lowest-income quintile had catastrophic health expenditures in 2002–03 (defined as expenditures of 20 percent or more of household available income after deduction of food expenditure). The proportion was higher (8 percent) in the second lowest quintile and then decreased with income to 5.7 percent in the highest quintile; the national average was 6.7 percent. When available income is defined as income above the poverty line, 17 percent spend more than 20 percent of their available income.

31. All amounts are in constant 2009 (January) prices.

32. Among those who used the SUS in the previous year, only 22 percent said that the service was bad or terrible.

33. Security and unemployment were 14 and 9 percent, respectively. As the study reports the relative ranking of different issues, the higher ranking of health as a key problem may reflect improvements in other areas rather than a worsening of the health system.

34. Although some studies point in this direction, they are difficult to reconcile with other studies that point to high levels of satisfaction. For instance, in the nationally representative PNAD, 16 percent of those obtaining care from the SUS said that it was "very good" and 64 percent that it was "good."

35. While many studies tend to focus on the public system, dissatisfaction with private plans is also high, but for different reasons. This suggests the need for effective oversight and regulation.

References

Abreu, D., C. Cesar, and E. Franca. 2007. "The Relationship between Deaths That Are Avoidable with Adequate Health Care and the Implementation of the Unified Health System in Brazil." *Revista Panamericana de Salud Pública* 21 (5): 282–91.

———. 2009. "Gender Differences in Avoidable Mortality in Brazil (1983–2005)." *Cadernos de Saúde Pública* 25 (12): 2672–82.

ANS (Agência Nacional de Saúde Suplementar). 2011. "Cadernos de informação da saúde suplementar." ANS, Brasilia, March.

Aquino, R., N. Oliveira, and M. Barreto. 2009. "Impact of Family Health Program on Infant Mortality in Brazilian Municipalities." *American Journal of Public Health* 99 (January): 87–93.

Axene, D., and S. McQuillian. 1999. *Analysis of Potentially Avoidable Inpatient Services.* Research Paper. Radnor, PA: Milliman and Robertson.

Barros, A., J. Bastos, and A. Damaso. 2011. "Catastrophic Spending on Health Care in Brazil: Private Health Insurance Does Not Seem to Be the Solution." *Cadernos de Saúde Pública* 27 (Suppl 2): S254–62.

Bertoldi, A., A. Barros, A. Camargo, P. Hallal, S. Vandoros, A. Wagner, and D. Ross-Degnan. 2011. "Household Expenditures for Medicines and the Role of Free Medicines in the Brazilian Public Health System." *American Journal of Public Health* 101 (5): 916–21.

Bertoldi, A., A. Barros, A. Wagner, D. Ross-Degnan, and P. Hallal. 2009. "Medicine Access and Utilization in a Population Covered by Primary Health Care in Brazil." *Health Policy* 89 (3): 295–302.

Bertoldi, A. D., A. P. Helfer, A. L. Camargo, N. U. Tavares, and P. Kanavos. 2012. "Is the Brazilian Pharmaceutical Policy Ensuring Population Access to Essential Medicines?" *Global Health* 8 (1): 6.

Bos, A. M., and H. Waters. 2008. "The Financial Protection Impact of the Public Health System and Private Insurance in Brazil." *CEPAL Review* 95 (August): 125–39.

Caminal, J., B. Starfield, and E. Sanchez. 2004. "The Role of Primary Care in Preventing Ambulatory Care Sensitive Conditions." *European Journal of Public Health* 14 (3): 246–51.

Campino, A. C. 2011. "Gastos catastróficos, iniquidade e proposta de reformulação do sistema de saúde." In *Brasil: A nova agenda social*, edited by E. Bacha and S. Schwartzman, 104–08. Rio de Janeiro: Long Term Care.

CNI (Confederação Nacional da Indústria). 2012. *Retratos da sociedade brasileira: Saúde pública*. Pesquisa CNI-IBOPE. Brasilia: CNI.

CNM (Confederação Nacional de Município). 2011. *Pesquisa da CNM sobre a demanda reprimida em saúde no Estado do Rio Grande do Sul*. Brasilia.

CONASS (Conselho Nacional de Secretários de Saúde). 2003: *A saúde na opinião dos brasileiros: Um estudo prospectivo*. Série Progestores. Brasilia: CONASS.

Couttolenc, B. 2011. "Taking Stock of Performance Reforms at the Sub-National Level in Brazil: Recent Performance Gains Achieved in the Health Sector, Hypotheses on Possible Drivers of Good and Bad Performance." Consultant report, World Bank, Washington, DC.

Couttolenc, B., L. Dias, and A. Nicolella. 2004. "Estudo de custos, eficiência e mecanismos de pagamento. Fase II: Eficiência e mecanismos de pagamento. Em busca da excelência: Fortalecendo o desempenho hospitalar no Brasil." Consultant report, World Bank, São Paulo.

CREMESP (Conselho Regional de Medicina do Estado de São Paulo). 2004. *Avaliação das condições de funcionamento dos hospitais e pronto-socorros, 2001–2003*. São Paulo: CREMESP.

Diniz, B., L. Servo, S. Piola, and M. Eirado. 2007. "Gasto das famílias com saúde no Brasil: Evolução e debate sobre gasto catastrófico." In *Gasto e consumo das famílias brasileiras contemporáneas*, edited by F. Faiger, L. Servo, T. Menezes, and S. Piola, 143–60. Brasilia: Instituto de Pesquisa Econômica Aplicada.

Dourado, I., V. Oliveira, R. Aquino, P. Bonolo, M. Lima-Costa, M. Medina, E. Mota, M. Turci, and J. Macinko. 2011. "Trends in Primary Health Care–Sensitive Conditions in Brazil: The Role of the Family Health Program (Project ICSAP-Brazil)." *Medical Care* 49 (6): 577–84.

Folha de São Paulo. 2012. "Insatisfação com a saúde sobe 11 pontos em um ano (2012)." *Folha de São Paulo*, January 25.

Garcia, L., M. Stivali, L. Santana, A. Pacheco Aurea, and L. Magalhaes. 2011. "Gastos das famílias brasilieras com medicamentos: Analyise dasa Pesquisas de Orcamentos

Familaries de 1995–1996, 2002–2003 e 2008–2009." Presentation at the Tenth Encontro Nacional da Economia de Saúde, Porto Alegre, October 26–28.

Gorgot, L., I. Santos, N. Valle, A. Matijasevich, A. Barros, and E. Albernaz. 2011. "Avoidable Deaths until 48 [Corrected] Months of Age among Children from the 2004 Pelotas Birth Cohort." *Revista de Saúde Pública* 45 (2): 334–42.

IBGE (Instituto Brasileiro de Geografia e Estatística). 2002. *Estatísticas da saúde: Assistência médico-sanitária (AMS) 2002.* Rio de Janeiro: IBGE. http://www.ibge. gov–br/home/estatistica/populacao/condicaodevida/ams/ams2002.pdf.

———. 2004. "Projeção da população do Brasil por sexo e idade para o período 1980–2050." Revised. Diretoria de Pesquisas, Coordenação de População e Indicadores Sociais, Gerência de Estudos e Análises da Dinâmica Demográfica, Rio de Janeiro.

———. 2006. *Estatísticas da saúde: Assistência médico-sanitária (AMS) 2005.* Rio de Janeiro: IBGE. http://www.ibge.gov.br/home/estatistica/populacao/condicaodevida/ ams/2005/ams2005.pdf.

———. 2009. *Indicadores sociodemográficos e de saúde no Brasil.* Rio de Janeiro: IBGE.

———. 2010. *Estatísticas da saúde: Assistência médico-sanitária (AMS) 2009.* Rio de Janeiro: IBGE.

———. Various years (1982–2009). *Pesquisa Nacional por Amostra de Domicílios (PNAD).* Brasilia: Ministério da Fazenda, Secretaria de Política Econômica.

IESS (Instituto de Estudos de Saúde Suplementar). 2011. "Pesquisa IESS/Datafolha aponta que o plan de saúde é uma necessidade e desejo do brasileiro." *Saúde Suplementar em Foco, Informativo Eletrônico* 2 (13).

IPEA (Instituto de Pesquisa Econômica Aplicada). 2011. *Sistema de indicadores de percepção social: Saúde.* Brasilia: IPEA.

Knaul, F., R. Wong, H. Arreola-Ornelas, and O. Mendez. 2011. "Household Catastrophic Health Expenditures: A Comparative Analysis of Twelve Latin American and Caribbean Countries." *Salud Pública Mexicana* 53 (Suppl. 2): S85–95.

La Forgia, G. M., and B. F. Couttolenc. 2008. *Hospital Performance in Brazil: In Search of Excellence.* Washington, DC: World Bank.

Legorreta, A., H. Chernicoff, J. Trinh, and R. Parker. 2004. "Diagnosis, Clinical Staging, and Treatment of Breast Cancer: A Retrospective Multiyear Study of a Large Controlled Population." *American Journal of Clinical Oncology* 27 (2): 185–90.

Macinko J. 2011. "A Preliminary Assessment of the Family Health Strategy (FHS) in Brazil." Consultant report, World Bank, Washington, DC.

Macinko, J., C. Almeida, and P. K. de Sá. 2007. "A Rapid Assessment Methodology for the Evaluation of Primary Care Organization and Performance in Brazil." *Health Policy and Planning* 22 (3): 167–77.

Macinko, J., F. Guanais, M. de Fatima, and M. de Souza. 2006. "Evaluation of the Impact of the Family Health Program on Infant Mortality in Brazil, 1990–2002." *Journal of Epidemiology and Community Health* 60 (1): 13–19.

Malta, D., E. Duarte, J. Escalante, M. Almeida, L. Sardinha, and E. Macario. 2010. "Avoidable Causes of Infant Mortality in Brazil, 1997–2006: Contributions to Performance Evaluation of the Unified National Health System." *Cadernos de Saúde Pública* 26 (3): 481–91.

Medici, A. 2003. *Family Spending on Health in Brazil: Some Indirect Evidence of the Regressive Nature of Public Spending in Health.* Technical Paper Series. Washington, DC: Inter-American Development Bank, Sustainable Development Department.

Ministry of Health. 2000. *Avaliação da implementação e funcionamento do Programa de Saúde da Família*. Ministério da Saúde, Secretaria de Assitencia da Saúde, Coordinação de Atenção Básica, Brasilia.

———. 2006. *Programa Nacional de Avaliação de Serviços de Saúde (PNASS): Resultado do processo avaliativo 2004–2006*. Brasilia: Ministério da Saúde.

———. 2008. *Saúde da família no Brasil: Uma análise de indicadores selecionados, 1998–2005/06*. Brasilia.

———. 2010a. "PCA-Tool." Ministério da Saúde, Brasilia.

———. 2010b. *Saúde Brasil 2009: Uma análise da situação de saúde e da agenda nacional e internacional de prioridades em saúde*. Brasilia.

Ministry of Health, SVS (Secretariat of Health Surveillance). 2011. "Sistema de informações sobre mortalidade." Ministério da Saúde, Brasilia.

Naves, O., and L. Silver. 2005. "Evaluation of Pharmaceutical Assistance in Public Primary Care in Brasilia, Brazil." *Revista de Saúde Pública* 39 (2): 223–30.

Nolte, E., and M. McKee. 2003. "Measuring the Health of Nations: Analysis of Mortality Amenable to Health Care." *British Medical Journal* 327 (7424): 1129.

O'Donnell, O., E. Van Doorslaer, A. Wagstaff, and M. Lindelow. 2008. *Analyzing Health Equity Using Household Survey Data: A Guide to Techniques and Their Implementation*. Washington, DC: World Bank.

OECD (Organisation for Economic Co-operation and Development). 2003. *OECD Reviews of Health Care Systems: Korea*. Paris: OECD.

———. 2011. *Health at a Glance 2011*. Paris: OECD.

Osorio, R., L. Servo, and S. Piola. 2011. "Unmet Health Care Needs in Brazil: An Investigation about the Reasons for Not Seeking Health Care." *Cien Saúde Colet* 16 (9): 3741–54.

Rocha, R. 2011. "Equidade no sistema de saúde brasileiro." Consultant report, World Bank, Washington, DC.

Rocha, R., and R. Soares. 2009. "Evaluating the Impact of Community-Based Health Interventions: Evidence from Brazil's Family Health Program." Discussion Paper 4119, IZA, Germany, Bonn.

Santos, I., A. Matijasevich, A. Barros, E. Albernaz, M. Domingues, and N. Valle. 2011. "Avoidable Deaths in the First Four Years of Life among Children in the 2004 Pelotas (Brazil) Birth Cohort Study." *Cadernos de Saúde Pública* 27 (Suppl. 2): S185–97.

Santos, J. Jr. 2006. "Avaliação médica: O consumo na medicina e a mercantilização da saúde." *Revista Brasileira de Coloproctologia* 26 (1): 70–85.

Santos, V., and S. Nitrini. 2004. "Prescription and Patient-Care Indicators in Health Care Services." *Revista de Saúde Pública* 38 (6): 819–26.

SES-MG (Secretaria de Estado da Saúde de Minas Gerais). 2005. "Caracterização da rede hospitalar do Sistema Único de Saúde em Minas Gerais: Estudos de políticas de saúde e de avaliação econômica do SUS-MG." Serviços Hospitalares 3, SES-MG, Belo Horizonte.

TCU (Tribunal de Contas da União). 2011. *Política nacional de atenção oncológica*. Brasília: TCU, Secretaria de Fiscalização e Avaliação de Programas de Governo.

Vali, F. 2001. *Access to Primary Care in New Jersey: Geographic Variation of Hospitalizations for Ambulatory Care Sensitive Conditions in 1995 and 1997*. Princeton, NJ: Health Research and Educational Trust of New Jersey.

Victora, C., E. Aquino, M. Leal, C. Monteiro, F. Barros, and C. Szwarcwald. 2011. "Saúde de mães e crianças no Brasil: Progressos e desafios." Série Saúde no Brasil 2. *thelancet. com* (May 9): 32–46.

Vieira, F. S. 2009. "Ministry of Health's Spending on Drugs: Program Trends from 2002 to 2007." *Revista de Saúde Publica* 43 (4): 674–81.

WHO (World Health Organization). 2008. *World Health Statistics 2008*. Geneva: WHO.

———. 2010. *World Health Statistics 2010*. Geneva: WHO.

World Bank. 1994. "The Organization, Delivery, and Financing of Health Care in Brazil: Agenda for the 1990s." Report 12655-BR, World Bank, Washington, DC.

———. 2002. "Brazil: Maternal and Child Health." Report 23811-BR, World Bank, Washington, DC.

———. 2010. *World Development Indicators*. Washington, DC: World Bank.

———. 2011. *World Development Indicators*. Washington, DC: World Bank.

Xu, K., D. B. Evans, K. Kawabata, R. Zeramdini, J. Klavus, and C. J. Murray. 2003. "Household Catastrophic Health Expenditure: A Multicountry Analysis." *Lancet* 362 (9378): 111–17.

CHAPTER 4

Conclusions

Over the last 20 years, Brazil has experienced impressive improvements in health outcomes, with dramatic reductions in child and infant mortality and increases in life expectancy. Equally important, geographic and socioeconomic disparities in outcomes have become far less pronounced. Needless to say, these achievements cannot be attributed solely to improvements in the health system. Indeed, the last 20 years have also seen continued urbanization, improved access to water and sanitation, and, at least in the last decade, rapid economic growth and lower income inequality.

Yet there are good reasons to believe that changes in the Unified Health System (Sistema Único de Saúde, SUS) have played an important role. The rapid expansion of primary care has changed the patterns of use, with a growing share of contacts taking place in health centers and other primary care facilities. The use of health services has risen, and the share of households reporting problems in accessing health care for financial reasons has declined. Moreover, this report has presented evidence that improvements in health can be attributed at least in part to the health system, with the expansion of primary care bringing about impressive reductions in mortality that is amenable to health care and in child mortality. In short, the SUS reforms have at least partially achieved the goals of universal and equitable access to health care.

Yet the report also has highlighted many challenges that remain in the SUS and the health system more broadly. Perhaps the most significant of these relate to the quality and coordination of care, gaps in coverage of primary care, barriers to accessing specialist and high-complexity care, and continued high reliance on private spending to finance health care. For instance, the expansion of primary care coverage has stagnated in recent years, and delays in the diagnosis and treatment of various forms of cancer reflect broader problems facing large segments of the population in trying to access specialist care. Moreover, quality is a concern throughout the system, with evidence that prenatal care is often not achieving its potential with regard to reducing maternal and infant deaths and that compliance with clinical protocols and approaches to improving quality are often weak. Partly as a result of remaining access and quality issues, Brazil still has significant ground to cover with respect to health outcomes; in spite of recent progress, the country still ranks around 95 out of 213 countries for both life expectancy and infant mortality.

At the same time, similar countries have achieved better health outcomes at similar or lower expenditure levels, suggesting that there is scope for improving the efficiency of Brazil's public health system.[1] Problems related to access and quality also contribute to the continued demand for private health plans and reliance on out-of-pocket expenditures to access care outside the SUS, undermining the goals of universality and equity. They are also the key factors explaining high and seemingly rising levels of public dissatisfaction with the health system.

These challenges are likely to get bigger in the future, as the health system has to deal with the consequences of a rapidly aging population and rising expectations. The ratio of elderly (over 65) to population in the productive ages in Brazil is expected to increase from 11 percent in 2005 to 49 percent in 2050, and life expectancy is likely to rise to 81 years over the same period (Gragnolati et al. 2011; IBGE 2004). Aging and lifestyle changes mean that a growing share of the burden of disease is the result of noncommunicable diseases.[2] These changes imply a need to move from a passive, curative pattern of care to one based on managing and controlling risk factors and modifying health habits, with implications for how the health system is organized, the skills that are needed, and the costs of delivering on the commitments of the SUS.[3] In summary, the rapid process of population aging presents the SUS—and the health sector in general—with a double challenge. First, it places greater financial pressure on the SUS, at a time when the system is facing mounting resistance to mobilizing additional resources under the current pattern of financing. Second, it creates pressure to reorganize the delivery of health care to deal more effectively with chronic diseases of the elderly.

Both the achievements and the challenges can be traced back, at least in part, to recent changes in how the health system is financed and organized. The establishment of the SUS represented an important break from the past. Yet, as noted in the report, the formal establishment of the SUS through the 1988 Constitution and subsequent legislation represents the culmination of a series of steps and movements toward universal coverage during the 1970s and 1980s. Moreover, while political policy and legislation are important, transforming the health system is a long process. Although 1988 was a critical juncture for health in Brazil, the impact of the reform is difficult to discern given the continuity with the past and the slow and gradual process of implementation.

Nonetheless, many of the structural reforms that were envisaged at the conception of the SUS have been achieved. In particular, there have been a dramatic decentralization of responsibilities for both financing and delivering health services; a deliberate reorientation of the health system toward primary care; a gradual shift of hospital services toward public sector providers; an increase in government spending on health, particularly in recent years; and establishment of robust and innovative mechanisms for social participation and intergovernmental coordination in the health sector. But the agenda is unfinished. Looking ahead, this report has highlighted five primary challenges.

Sustaining Improvements in Access to Health Care

The report has described the rapid and impressive expansion of access to primary care in Brazil and the impact that this expansion has had on the use of health services and health outcomes. Yet costs, lack of qualified staff, and other factors have slowed the pace of expansion in recent years, with the Family Health Strategy (ESF) reaching 50 percent of the population. As Brazil continues its effort to fill these gaps, parallel efforts will be needed to improve the quality of primary care. However, diverse models of primary care are currently in use, and it will be important to reach some consensus on their relative merits (and costs).

While the path for sustaining improvements in the coverage of primary care is relatively clear, efforts to achieve true "integrality" of care are likely to meet with more challenges. Problems with coordination of care and access to specialist, diagnostic, and hospital services have multiple and complex causes, including lack of infrastructure and human resource capacity, inadequate payment rates (incentives) for some procedures, complex contracting arrangements with private sector providers, and weak referral and counterreferral systems. Many initiatives are under way to address these challenges: investment and upgrading of capacity, review of payment rates, implementation of clinical guidelines, investment in systems for referrals and electronic medical records, and so forth. In most cases (with the possible exception of large metropolitan areas), these reforms require effective coordination across municipalities and are best implemented in the context of regional health care networks. Even then, they are complex and expensive reforms that need to be sequenced appropriately and coordinated. Many important lessons can be learned from the Organisation for Economic Co-operation and Development (OECD) and other middle-income countries in this regard. It will also be important to establish mechanisms for monitoring and evaluating reforms in Brazil and for sharing experiences across states and municipalities so that lessons are learned along the way.

As part of this process, it will be important to address the lack of integration between the SUS and the private sector and to define their roles clearly. Competition and lack of coordination between the two sectors result in duplications of efforts and resources, conflicts over who should pay for what, and difficulty in addressing systemwide problems. Under the SUS, an important step was taken in establishing a regulatory framework, albeit one with gaps and unresolved issues. But coordination between the two sectors remains very weak, and inconsistencies between SUS basic legislation, which confers a marginal role on the private sector, and the existence of a strong dynamic private sector need to be reconciled.

Improving Efficiency and Quality of Health Care Services

The report has highlighted challenges pertaining to quality and efficiency in the delivery of some services as well as important capacity gaps in some specialist and high-complexity areas. The SUS reforms did not include specific goals or targets in relation to how service delivery was to be organized, but the public sector was expected to take on an increasingly important role in the delivery of health services. This is what has happened, in particular in the hospital sector.

Yet in the face of persistent concerns about efficiency and quality, many states and municipalities are experimenting with new models for providing services. For instance, São Paulo has pioneered the contracting of hospital services from nonprofit organizations (*organizações sociais*). Rio de Janeiro is using a similar approach for primary care, and many other states and municipalities are following suit. While these contracting arrangements tend to be very collaborative in nature, they require explicit performance standards and government capacity to monitor and enforce contracts—requirements that put significant new demands on the state and municipal health secretariats.

In many parts of Brazil there is also increased experimentation with public-private partnerships, in both the construction and the management of public facilities. For instance, Bahia recently implemented a public-private partnership for the Hospital do Subúrbio in Salvador. Such partnerships can bring important benefits to the health sector, but only if the government chooses the right projects and has the capacity to design, monitor, and enforce contracts.

Separate from new models for contracting or partnering with the private sector, both the federal Ministry of Health and local governments are working on approaches to stimulate improvements in efficiency and quality by setting more explicit standards for services and creating financial incentives for providers. For instance, the Ministry of Health is about to roll out a National Program for Improvement of Access and Quality in Primary Care (Programa Nacional de Melhoria do Acesso e da Qualidade da Atenção Básica, PMAQ), which will define performance indicators and targets and provide incentives for municipalities to achieve these targets. New modalities for contracts between the federal government and regional health care networks (tripartite agreements between federal, state, and municipal governments) also entail an increased focus on results.[4]

The establishment of new contracting models will provide an opportunity to change how providers are financed and how levels of government relate to one another. However, outside of these experiences, an important factor that contributes to inefficiency and poor quality is the weakness of current mechanisms for paying providers. Even when an originally adequate design has been adopted, as with the inpatient care information and billing system of the SUS (*autorização de internação hospitalar*, AIH), distortions have accumulated; current payment methods do not provide appropriate incentives to service providers. Correcting existing distortions and adopting methods that give providers clear incentives to contain costs and improve quality will make more effective use of available resources and further improve the performance of the health system.

However, payment reform will have to go hand-in-hand with measures to increase the financial and managerial autonomy of hospitals if the payment-related incentives are to have an impact on performance.

Overall, Brazil has undertaken extensive experimentation with approaches to improve efficiency and quality in service delivery. Many of these hold promise, but there clearly are no silver bullets. Moreover, in many cases, implementation of reforms has been piecemeal and on a limited scale. It will be important to ensure that these experiences are evaluated systematically and that the lessons from these evaluations are shared widely among stakeholders in Brazil. In some areas, meaningful reforms will require strong federal leadership. This is the case, for instance, with provider payment reform and implies the need for significant changes from current modalities for financing medium- and high-complexity services. Similarly, federal initiatives such as PMAQ, with national support for coordination and implementation, robust monitoring and reporting arrangements, and rigorous evaluation, can have a profound impact on the quality of primary care. The ongoing efforts to establish regional networks may provide opportunities for establishing similar initiatives to improve the efficiency and quality of specialist and hospital services.

Clarifying Roles and Relationships across Levels of Government

Decentralization of the health sector has expanded the role of both municipalities and states in the financing and delivery of health services. This has brought many benefits, such as increased accountability, tailoring of the system to local needs, coordination with other public services, and so forth. Yet many municipalities lack the scale and technical capacity to manage a health system involving all levels of care and complex support services, and many states have not played the requisite role in coordination and support. Moreover, even with a growing share of municipal spending allocated to health, complementary financing by the state and federal governments is needed, both to achieve equity and to promote higher-level goals and objectives. A well-functioning system will depend on effective coordination and collaboration across municipalities, in particular when it comes to specialist and high-complexity services, referral systems, and medical logistics (for example, patients and medical supplies). It will also depend on robust institutions and approaches for contracting and financing across levels of government.

In both of these areas, Brazil has made significant strides in recent years, with new legislation to support the establishment of regional networks (comprising several municipalities), a framework for contracting between federal government and health regions, and institutional mechanisms for coordinating between municipalities, states, and federal government. However, implementation of this legislation will inevitably raise many political and practical challenges relating to the process of regional planning, management, and coordination of "shared" services, how to finance investments in systems and capacity to support regional networks, how to share financing responsibilities across levels of government, and so forth. Different states will proceed at different speeds, and it will be important to study and learn from the early adopters.

Determining the Right Level of Health Spending and Improving Efficiency

Although there is continued pressure from the health establishment to increase public health funding to allow the SUS to fulfill its mandate, a key question is whether a higher level of public financing is needed at all. That is, is the level of public spending on health in Brazil adequate, in relation both to SUS constitutional responsibilities and to expectations of the population? The report has presented data showing that spending increased significantly over the last 20 years in absolute terms (and to a lesser extent as a share of gross domestic product, GDP). However, the growth in spending was slower than in many other middle- and high-income countries, in particular, those that have experienced a rapid expansion in coverage (for example, the Republic of Korea, South Africa, Thailand, and Turkey). Moreover, the increase in spending did not keep up with the rapid expansion of the system and the volume of services provided, in particular, if cost increases associated with the introduction of new drugs and procedures are also considered.

More government spending on health would undoubtedly help to finance more health system resources (facilities, equipment, staff), medical supplies, and services. Yet the report has shown that the lack of resources and supplies often is not a binding constraint to improving access and quality. For instance, La Forgia and Couttolenc (2008) found that hospitals operate at a high level of inefficiency and that the average Brazilian hospital could produce three times its current output with the same amount of inputs if it were as efficient as the most efficient hospitals. Hospital beds and operating theaters are largely underused, and expensive diagnostic equipment is oversupplied in many regions. And at least to some extent, problems of access to diagnostic and specialist care have more to do with how the health system is organized (weak management, lack of functioning referral systems) than with a lack of resources per se.

Hence, although the debate over whether the public system is "adequately" or "sufficiently" funded has raged since before its foundation, there is no clear and scientific way to determine whether this is the case. In Brazil, the health system clearly could produce more health services and better health outcomes with the same level of resources if it were more efficient. For instance, significant gains could be achieved by aligning hospital capacity more closely with need, enhancing technical efficiency of hospitals through better management and incentives, reducing waste and misuse of funds, and so forth. Gains could also be realized through improved prioritization in the allocation of government spending (a shift toward services and interventions that are more cost-effective), which in turn would require a more robust process for making decisions about the introduction and management of existing and new technologies (drugs and procedures). There are no simple solutions for dealing with these issues, but there is a wealth of international experience on which to draw.

At the same time, even with improvements in efficiency, spending pressures are unlikely to abate in coming decades. As a share of GDP, government spending on health in Brazil (around 4.5 percent) is less than half the OECD average. In part, the higher government spending in many OECD countries is explained by the fact that health is an inherently labor-intensive sector, and the relative cost of health services tends to rise as GDP grows. But it is also explained by differences in demographics and the coverage and quality of services provided.

As Brazil continues to grow and develop, the combination of unmet need in both primary and specialist care, the introduction of new technology (drugs and procedures), growing demand for health care associated with noncommunicable diseases, and higher use associated with an aging population is likely to put significant pressure on public health spending in the decades to come. As in other advanced health systems around the world, it will be essential to enhance efficiency and improve prioritization, but it will also be important to prepare for significant and sustained increases in government health spending and put in place mechanisms for managing the cost pressures that are already evident in the system. This is likely to include more robust systems for assessing and managing the introduction and use of new technologies in the form of hardware, procedures, and pharmaceuticals.

Conducting More and Better Health System Monitoring and Research

Brazil has a strong tradition of evidence-based policy making in the health sector and a vibrant health research community. The report has highlighted the need to build on these strengths to support continued health system reform. For instance, although vast amounts of administrative data on health outcomes, delivery of health services, and health financing are publicly available, problems often plague the quality of data, consistency of definitions, and structure of data over time and space. This makes it difficult to benchmark performance over time, across space, and internationally in some areas. Data are missing on many important dimensions of performance, including waiting times for elective procedures, quality of chronic disease care, and survival rates for specific conditions such as cancer and heart attacks. Data on these types of indicators have played a very important role in understanding and addressing health system challenges in OECD countries and will gain importance as Brazil grapples with issues relating to access, quality, and coordination of care. Despite the valid methodological concerns that have been raised, the Ministry of Health's initiative to define a new set of indicators for monitoring and benchmarking performance (Índice de Desempenho do SUS, SUS Performance Indicator, IDSUS) represents an important step toward addressing this gap.

Beyond the monitoring of health system performance, the report has highlighted several areas where in-depth research is warranted. What are the costs and relative merits of different primary health care models? What are the impacts of the approaches to improving quality and improving efficiency that are being considered? What are the advantages and risks associated with public contracting of health care from nonprofit providers? How can the high levels of out-of-pocket spending on medicines be reduced? How does the establishment of regional networks affect the structure, organization, and performance of local health systems? How do different models of health system governance and financing, including across levels of government, affect the performance of the system? These are merely some of the questions that rigorous research and evaluation, based on strong partnerships between policy makers and the research community, can help answer and, in that way, contribute to making the Brazilian health system more efficient, effective, and equitable.

Notes

1. Ranking is based on the most recent data in the World Bank, World Development Indicators database.

2. Noncommunicable diseases already account for about two-thirds of the burden of disease in Brazil, compared with 24 percent from communicable diseases and 10 percent from injuries.

3. For instance, a recent study by the Instituto de Pesquisa Econômica Aplicada found that 71 percent of Brazilian municipalities did not have any institution for elder care and that existing institutions—two-thirds of which were not-for-profit organizations— cared for only 0.5 percent of the elderly population (IPEA 2011).

4. The model is based on the organizational contract for public action in health (*contrato organizativo da acão pública da saúde*).

References

Gragnolati, M., O. H. Jorgensen, R. Rocha, and A. Fruttero. 2011. *Getting Old in an Older Brazil: Implications of Population Aging on Economic Growth, Poverty Reduction, Public Finance, and Service Delivery*. Directions in Development Series. Washington, DC: World Bank.

IBGE (Instituto Brasileiro de Geografia e Estatística). 2004. "Projeção da população do Brasil por sexo e idade para o período 1980–2050." IBGE, Diretoria de Pesquisas, Coordenação de População e Indicadores Sociais, Gerência de Estudos e Análises da Dinâmica Demográfica, Rio de Janeiro.

IPEA (Instituto de Pesquisa Econômica Aplicada). 2011. "Condições de funcionamento e infraestrutura das instituições de longa permanência para idosos no Brasil." Comunicados IPEA 93, Série Eixos do Desenvolvimento Brasileiro, IPEA, Brasilia.

La Forgia, G., and B. Couttolenc. 2008. *Hospital Performance in Brazil: In Search of Excellence*. Washington, DC: World Bank.

Environmental Benefits Statement

The World Bank is committed to reducing its environmental footprint. In support of this commitment, the Office of the Publisher leverages electronic publishing options and print-on-demand technology, which is located in regional hubs worldwide. Together, these initiatives enable print runs to be lowered and shipping distances decreased, resulting in reduced paper consumption, chemical use, greenhouse gas emissions, and waste.

The Office of the Publisher follows the recommended standards for paper use set by the Green Press Initiative. Whenever possible, books are printed on 50% to 100% postconsumer recycled paper, and at least 50% of the fiber in our book paper is either unbleached or bleached using Totally Chlorine Free (TCF), Processed Chlorine Free (PCF), or Enhanced Elemental Chlorine Free (EECF) processes.

More information about the Bank's environmental philosophy can be found at http://crinfo.worldbank.org/crinfo/environmental_responsibility/index.html.

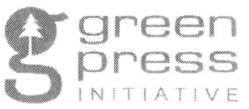